UNDEFEATED

FROM TRAGEDY TO TRIUMPH

MARC BUONICONTI

with George Abaunza, PhD, and Mark Vancil

A POST HILL PRESS BOOK

Undefeated:
From Tragedy to Triumph
© 2017 by Marc Buoniconti
All Rights Reserved

ISBN: 978-1-68261-457-0
ISBN (eBook): 978-1-68261-458-7

Cover Design by Ryan Truso
Interior Design and Composition by Greg Johnson/Textbook Perfect

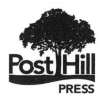

Post Hill Press
New York • Nashville
posthillpress.com

Published in the United States of America

I dedicate this book to my parents,
Terry and Nick Buoniconti,
both of whom I love very much!!

They gave me life 50 years ago,
and the strength to be born again in 1985
after my life-threatening injury.
They are the foundation upon which
I continue to fight for a cure for paralysis
and to help change the world!

A Special Thanks

I'd like to give my special thanks to my co-writers,
George Abaunza, PhD, and Mark Vancil,
and co-editors, Stephanie Sayfie Aagaard, Priscilla Marrero,
Suzanne M. Sayfie, and Sherida Yoder, PhD.

I could not have written this book without them.

TABLE OF CONTENTS

Part II INTO THE DEEP

PART III THE RISING

FOREWORD

Many years ago, I was invited to visit the spinal cord injury wing of a Boston hospital. I declined, saying, "I don't think I can take it; as an active outdoorsman I have an aversion to those kind of injuries. I can't imagine being immobilized."

My host persisted.

"You really should see these people," he said. "They know you love rock climbing, running rivers, backpacking, skiing. You'll learn a lot from them."

I went, reluctantly, and the first patient I met was doing wheelies in her wheelchair. She had been hurt in a diving accident but she was still gung ho and upbeat. So was the guy paralyzed in a motorcycle accident. Ditto the skier. Yes, they were all living differently than they had been a few years earlier, but they had not given up on life.

It was the beginning of a personal fascination with, and a commitment to people with spinal cord injuries and the science of trying to advance progress toward a cure.

My involvement went to a new level when I became friendly with the Buoniconti family. The father, Nick, was a generational contemporary. We're the same age, and I had watched his playing days with awe and admiration, first as an All-American at Notre Dame, then as an All-Pro linebacker with the fabled unbeaten Miami Dolphins.

When Marc was gravely hurt playing football for The Citadel, I read the accounts of the family rushing to his side and Nick vowing to find a cure for spinal cord injuries.

It was so much more than an emotional outburst. It was the beginning of The Miami Project to Cure Paralysis, a state-of-the-art laboratory, clinic, and rehabilitation center that has advanced the knowledge and treatment of spinal cord injuries far down the field.

Dr. Barth Green and his associates have given the world and all the families with spinal cord injury concerns more than clinical trials of exciting new cell therapy techniques, drugs, surgeries, advanced rehabilitation practices, and compassion, always compassion.

They have given us hope.

In the process, the Buoniconti family has given something else just as important, just as precious. They have given us all lessons in how to be a family. How to love one another even when the strain is great, how to stay a family even when the structure changes, how to have a common goal and pursue it with such passion and commitment to excellence that it becomes a force unto itself.

At the center of all this is Marc, one of the bravest, most decent and giving people I know. He was injured as a young man playing a game he loved. His life has been a struggle through every waking moment from that time forward. Yet he refuses to accept that constant condition as a burden. It has become for him a way of life and, more important, an opportunity to change the world of spinal cord injury.

This is his story.

Read it and weep, cheer, reflect, and come away knowing you've been in the presence of a young man with a power no paralyzed limb could diminish.

Read it and hope that you could be so brave.

Read it and stand, as Marc cannot, and cheer him on.

–Tom Brokaw

INTRODUCTION

I can't begin to relate the high regard I have for the Buoniconti family. I am in awe of their indestructible bond and the love they have for each other. Nick and Marc's phenomenal father/son relationship is one I can relate to, having shared a similar bond with my father, Joseph, a dedicated family man and compassionate individual whom I loved and respected at the highest level.

For the past thirty-three years, the Buoniconti father/son team has been passionately involved in supporting and directing a world-renowned research facility, The Miami Project to Cure Paralysis, dedicated to finding a cure for paralysis. I was introduced to this most worthy cause some years ago at the Great Sports Legends Dinner in New York City, and since that day I have pledged to Stand Up for Those Who Can't. I have been the presenting sponsor of the New York Dinner and made a $2.2 million gift to The Buoniconti Fund as well a $1 million donation at The Buoniconti Fund's Destination Fashion event in Miami.

I was pleased to join this father/son team again in our mission to find a cure for paralysis. I stood up at the Great Sports Legends Dinner to commit another $1 million in celebration of their twenty-fifth anniversary of the Dinner as well as the creation of this incredible book.

My indefatigable hope is that Marc and others who are paralyzed will someday be able to step out of their wheelchairs and walk again. Nothing would give me greater pleasure than to stand alongside my friend, Marc, when he takes those first momentous steps.

–Stewart Rahr*

*Stewart Rahr became a supporter of The Buoniconti Fund when he was the President, CEO, and sole owner of Kinray, the largest privately held pharmaceutical/generic distributor in the world. Mr. Rahr's success story has been over a forty-year

journey, back to when he took the reins of Kinray Pharmacy from his father, Joseph. The company since has grown from five employees and less than $1 million in annual revenue to more than 1,000 employees and more than $5 billion in annual income. Mr. Rahr has since sold the company and has been a loyal and generous contributor to many charities. His philanthropy has benefited hundreds of organizations, including The Buoniconti Fund to Cure Paralysis, which holds a special place in his heart.

Prologue

Third and One

Few of us know in advance the moment that changes our lives. It's only in retrospect that we identify a crucial twist embraced, or avoided. We operate largely without a map, turning right or left at the next intersection on the basis of experience, speculation, or random curiosity. The "choices" are often unconscious, and beyond our awareness. We feel our way through life's contours.

Fate is nothing more than the public performance of accumulated decisions. Turning left to avoid a life-threatening accident has less to do with the instinctive action than the life experiences up to that moment in time. Do we take implied consequences "like a man," or do we confront whatever is in front of us with guile, grit, and cunning?

Life is a series of third-and-one situations, though we often aren't aware of the significance one way or another. That's the beauty and the curse of sports. The moments present themselves on the basis of a clock, the score, distance, preparation, and strategy, all of which are subject to dozens of nuances. In football, the object of the game is to move the ball downfield to score against the other team's defense. The offensive team has four downs to move ten yards to gain another four downs. Each play is important, but games turn on third down. If the offensive team fails to gain another first down, then it's forced to turn the ball over to the opponent. On third down with a yard to go, everyone digs in a little deeper.

For most people that doesn't mean a thing. But for a football player, it's the difference between success and failure. For the offense, it's the opportunity to extend the possession. For the defense, it's a chance to stop the drive. There are no illusions. It's one side trying to impose its will on the other. The stakes are straightforward and self-evident to every player, coach, and fan.

In effect, the essence of the game is compressed into a single play. A more intense new rush of adrenaline and bravado rises to the surface. The crowd becomes louder because the moment creates the same chemical reaction in them. The noise a player hears, even inside a small domed stadium with the ground covered in artificial turf, is more of a low rumble. It's the vibration of sound more than anything familiar or discernible. Heart rates rise, focus narrows.

I lived for those moments. I thrived on the challenge, the extra degree of difficulty. It wasn't just on the football field. I lived my life in that context, pushing limits, eager to see what was around the next corner, or where I might find myself after one test or another. Dive deep into the ocean for two or three minutes without oxygen? I can do that. Climb forty feet to the top of a tree and jump off executing a flip into a narrow canal? No problem. Defy rules designed to limit very broad ideas of fun? Of course, why conform when not conforming provides so much entertainment? Test the limits of drugs and alcohol, skip school, hang out with dangerous dudes, buy drugs in the neighborhoods those guys did business in, even when some of those "friends" ended up dead, or in penitentiaries? Come on, danger is part of the fun, man.

What looked out of control to others was a confirmation of control to me. I wasn't dead. I wasn't in jail. I was in college, the starting linebacker for a hard-ass military school devoid of females and full of hard-ass guys.

What's going to happen next? Some people try to control life. Not me. You might as well try to grab a handful of air. What could be more inspiring than the confrontation directly in front of you?

On third-and-one it all comes together. At the most basic level, it captures the nature of the game and to one degree or another life itself. Who's tougher? Who's smarter? Who's more talented? Who wants it more? Who's willing to endure more pain? Who can feel the rhythm of a game, the sway of momentum? Who can focus in so narrowly that figuring out what the opponent will do next is reduced from speculation to near certainty?

In less than ten seconds it all plays out and the questions are answered. That's the allure of sports. There is instant gratification. Every decision is resolved almost immediately. Life is different that way. A decision made without a second thought can change the course of a life a week later.

As the middle linebacker, my eyes widened as I keyed on the center. When the center lunged toward me as he snapped the ball, his movements told me all I needed to know. I stepped to my left brushing him aside and locked in on the ball. There is almost no perception of sound. The arms and legs are those of people, but in the moment they are obstacles to be avoided, or to be shoved aside in pursuit of the ball.

I was running close to full speed when the quarterback flipped the ball to a low-slung running back with thick powerful legs. He knew what I knew: It was third-and-one.

Otherwise, we had nothing in common. He was African-American with a dark history born of a rough, dangerous childhood in a neighborhood that mirrored his experience. From the porch of the small house he grew up in, the running back watched as his father was shot to death in broad daylight in the front yard.

In my life, the sun shined nearly every day. I loved my childhood, my siblings, and my parents. Our house was on a canal with tall trees. We had our own swimming pool, a large lawn to play football, and a basketball court. My dad was a celebrity with trophies and championship rings from his life in professional football. My mother was a loving woman every bit as strong as my dad. I had everything that was important to a healthy, positive life.

But in that moment, there was no history. We were two people with a singular mission. Mine was the exact opposite of his. He needed the yard. Three feet. I needed to stop him.

The running back swung wide, gaining speed when one of my teammates flew into his legs. The running back flipped into the air. Instinctively I calculated where I had to slam into the hurtling body to stop his momentum. I took one final step in an all-out sprint, then dove straight toward the impact zone. I saw the number 20 upside down on his uniform. With the running back's head nearly touching the ground and his legs straight up in the air, he lunged forward toward the first down, grasping for every inch.

I was *locked* in and loaded. I flew toward the target with every ounce of force I could generate.

Nothing about the moment was unusual or out of character with the tone and tenor of my life. All the daring and risky behavior came together thanks in part to an innate arrogance long cultivated by successfully navigating the consequences of a life lived free, and reckless.

Then, in an instant, it was over.

I never felt a thing.

* * *

DAD: October 26, 1985, was a Saturday. My wife, Terry, and I were sitting on the terrace of my Notre Dame roommate Richard Catenacci's Hunterdon County, NJ, farmhouse. Richard's property extended over twenty-five or thirty acres and included a pond. Over the years he'd restored the house that looked out over the valley—just spectacular. We were kind of pinching ourselves. We had known one another and remained best friends for more than twenty-five years. We were doing well.

Richard was the managing partner in the biggest law firm in New Jersey. I had three children in college, and they were doing great. As we sat there we were saying, "How lucky can we be? How lucky can we be? Here we are. I'm doing well. You're doing well. We're drinking champagne, celebrating on one of the most phenomenal fall afternoons."

It was remarkable.

* * *

Whose arm is that?

Bodies were scattered around me. The arm didn't appear to go with any of them.

My body tingled. It wasn't pain so much as an absence of feeling. With little success, and even that diminishing I gasped to catch my breath. Seconds passed. Reality flooded in. I consciously confronted my emotions. If I panicked, I'd die.

The trainer reached me first. He peered into my eyes. His calm demeanor was betrayed by the horror on his face. He could only imagine what he couldn't see.

I mouthed three words: "I can't move." I knew what had happened. Still, the recognition was overwhelming. I didn't need a diagnosis. It was written on the faces of everyone around me.

I lay on the artificial turf in a small domed stadium, somewhere between life and death, for thirty minutes. How I survived is unknown, a miracle inside a nightmare.

I recall only one thought: don't panic.

The arm was mine.

Part I

OFF THE CHAIN

Chapter I

A Rebel in Child's Clothing

When does a life story begin? There are monumental moments that signal beginnings; some we choose and some chosen for us. A few of them define us. Others test what we believe to be essential and meaningful.

My life was transformed by one of those moments, a specific point in time from which a new life emerged.

Decisions and choices are actions that have repercussions. Although we often sense that only the monumental moments define us, transformation can be triggered by an ordinary choice. It can happen in an instant, and it can appear to have no connection to the future.

Choosing often has as many consequences as not choosing at all. Both are actions, even the seemingly inconsequential and mundane options that beget future events.

What is the extent of our agency? How much control over our lives do we have? How many neurosurgeons grow up in a house full of plumbers? Was it my idea to play football? Was the intensity and drive innate, or was it learned amid unique conditions?

To what extent do we get to choose? I was young, physically gifted, mentally prepared, and endowed with a family history that came with expectations, defined by ideas such as sacrifice, toughness, and personal responsibility. My brother was the starting linebacker for Duke University; our father was acknowledged as one of the greatest players in the history of professional football. I knew what excellence looked like. I knew the difference between commitment and contentment. I knew the game. And I knew how to define myself inside its white lines.

Our existence is based on an ideal. We have the illusion of free choice and full autonomy. Yet we are emotional beings uniquely predisposed to manipulation. When we choose, do we understand the difference between what we want and why we want it? Is it a deep need for acceptance that drives one decision at the expense of another? Is the act of rebelling against authority about me or, about the authority figure?

In my case, a series of moments isolated the person I had been from the person I was destined to become. The grand irony is it took the former to keep the latter alive.

I love to daydream. Even as a child, I would occupy myself for hours focusing on whatever was passing through my mind, except, of course, the future. I never spent much time thinking about anything beyond the next moment because there was always too much fun to be had in the present, even with the considerable bumps in the road that accrue to a nonconforming child.

Like love and trouble, life's changes appear to come slowly before arriving all at once. Growing up the only thing I knew about change is that it always presented a brand-new adventure.

My earliest memories are of our house in Randolph, MA, about fifteen miles south of Boston. By 1969, my dad had played seven seasons of professional football for the Boston Patriots in the American Football League. Even as a toddler, I can recall my sister Gina, my brother Nicky, and me swinging on the neighbors' swing set singing "Proud Mary" by Creedence Clearwater Revival and "Spinning Wheel" by Blood, Sweat & Tears. It's easy to remember when I heard music for the first time. Music touched my soul and offered a means of escape—perfect for my daydreaming. Music would continue to bring meaning throughout my life, serving as a chronology with each genre marking the different periods.

By the end of 1969, our family uprooted and headed to South Florida. The Miami Dolphins were a fledgling expansion NFL team. Ownership offered my father a deal he couldn't refuse. Suddenly and quite unexpectedly, Miami was our new home. We lived in a small community of townhouses called The Villas, in the Pinecrest area of South Dade. As my mom tells the story, the excitement started on the day we arrived. The three of us kids, fresh from New England, and without one swimming lesson between us, jumped into the swimming pool, clothes and all. As we sank to the bottom, in went my mother—also fully dressed—to pluck us out one by one. Welcome to Miami!

Several of the Dolphins players lived at The Villas, which made it a great playground. Every day, I ran to each of the neighbors, who loaded me up with cookies, candy, and whatever assorted goodies were within arm's reach. It got to a point where I had so many snacks during the day that I wouldn't eat my dinner. My mom adopted an ingenious, yet deceitful tactic. She greeted me one morning with a string attached to a cardboard sign. She proceeded to hang it around my neck.

"What is it, Mommy?"

"It's a sign."

"What does it say?"

"It says that you're a good boy."

I was so proud that I ran around the complex showing everybody my sign. As it turned out, the sign actually said, "Please don't feed me." Two things resulted from that episode. First, I stopped receiving the treats. And second, I figured out that being a good boy doesn't necessarily lead to reward. It was a foreshadowing of things to come.

My first recollection of school was kindergarten at Kendall Academy. The days were filled with arts and crafts, playing outside, swimming, and just all-around good fun. Then came one of those defining moments that become seared into our memory. The teacher stood in front of the class and said something unbelievable.

"If you complete this important project," she announced, "you will get a chance to fly in a spaceship."

I was so excited. To the best of my ability, I completed the project. I wanted to go on a spaceship! This was 1971. Just two years earlier

America landed the first humans on the moon. Every kid in the country wanted to be an astronaut. This was my chance! The day came for our work to be reviewed by the teacher.

Amazingly, she said everyone completed the task. It was thrilling. All I knew was that I was going on a spaceship. I didn't care whether any of my schoolmates were joining me. Then came the disappointment. Our teacher unveiled a drawing of a spaceship on the wall. One by one she wrote our names on pieces of paper, pinning them onto the spaceship. It was all a hoax! All my hopes and dreams of being an astronaut were shot down by a calculated swoop of brainwashing and behavior modification.

From that point on, I saw school as a place where adults manipulated children. Teachers were nothing more than puppet masters. For me, school went downhill from there, though it was a rounding error in terms of the childhood fun meter. Growing up in Miami in the 1970s was great.

By the time I entered first grade in 1972, the Miami Dolphins was on the verge of becoming one of the most iconic teams in the history of professional sports, recording the league's only undefeated season and winning the Super Bowl that season and the next. For the most part, though, the pomp was lost on a six-year-old. I had a sense that my father was different, but the idea of his celebrity and fame didn't resonate with me until much later, especially since my Dad worked during the offseason, as did most of the other players back then.

During the season, he would load Nicky and me into his green Cadillac and take us to the Orange Bowl on Saturdays for the walk-through—a dress rehearsal for Sunday games. The Orange Bowl, built in 1937, was the largest stadium in the state of Florida at the time. It was located just west of downtown in Little Havana. To my brother and me, though, it was the largest playground in the world.

We ran around the field, or slipped into the locker room to steal rolls of white tape the players used to wrap their ankles, wrists, and fingers. The stadium was one big erector set to a kid. There was so much to explore and we had free rein. The entire scene was exciting. We held the ball while the Dolphins kicker, Garo Yepremian, practiced field goals. We watched from one end of the field as coach Don

Shula took the team through plays at the other end. It was like going to the office with your father, except this one had seats for seventy-five thousand people.

There weren't a lot of other kids because my dad was one of the older players on the team. I ran around with Coach Shula's sons, David and Michael. Many years later, Michael and I were teammates at Miami's Christopher Columbus High School. No one worried about us because there wasn't anything to worry about back then. Dick Anderson, an All-Pro safety, was one of our neighbors. Bill Stanfill, an All-Pro defensive end, used to offer us "candy," which was actually chewing tobacco. I remember attending a golf tournament in Marco Island, Florida, one summer. My mom had Nicky and me dressed up for a poolside cocktail party. Two Dolphins players decided it would be fun to throw us into the pool. It was just men being men, and boys being boys. The players thought it was hilarious. Not my mom. Still, it felt as though we were part of a big family in a way that probably isn't possible in professional sports today.

Although she didn't appreciate the off-the-field shenanigans, when it came to the game, she was a fanatic. She knew the intricacies of professional football better than most men. When the team was on the road, the only thing we were concerned about was my mother making it through the telecast. No one could watch the game in the same room as her. She'd have a cigarette in one hand, a drink in the other, and would scream and yell like she was standing on the sidelines. I don't think my mother ever worried about my father being injured. He seemed indestructible. Like him, she was only interested in the Dolphins winning.

Throughout my dad's football career, he was considered small for a middle linebacker. Heck, at 5-foot-11 and 220 pounds he would be considered small for a safety today. I remember him coming home after games with various injuries—a busted hand in a plaster cast, for example. Another time, I was probably six or seven years old and my dad was sitting on the couch. I was surprised to see him, and I yelled "Dad!" as I ran into the room to leap onto his lap. As I flew through the air he put up his forearm so that I wouldn't land anywhere near him. All I heard from him was, "Oh, my ribs. My ribs." My dad was never seriously injured despite playing a position that was predicated on hitting people on just about every play. He played fifteen years and only missed part of one season due to injury. The game was every bit as brutal then as it is now. In some ways, it was even more so because of the equipment, or lack of it, and the often overlooked rough play. But my dad used his intellect and quickness to make plays and avoid injury.

He was also responsible for making my first year of grade school more positive than all other years of grade school combined. My teacher at Epiphany Catholic School, Sister Estelle, was a huge Dolphins fan. She gave me the treatment. She spoiled me to death. Sometimes my mother would come to pick me up from school, and I'd be at the convent eating cookies and hanging out with the nuns. It was a great year all around.

After a couple years, we moved from The Villas into a house in the Pinecrest neighborhood full of kids. This was an upper-middle-class area, a few miles south of downtown Miami, just east of US 1. A tourist attraction, the Parrot Jungle, isn't far from where I grew up. It's still a beautiful area. Most of the homes were built in the 1950s, 1960s, and early 1970s, on half-acre to three-quarter-acre lots.

We lived in a single-story home with a small yard and a two-car garage on a busy corner of a short street. One day my brother and I are pushing toy cars from one side of the street to the other. It is the kind of creative, make-up fun kids don't have these days. We push the cars across the street, then run to the other side and do it over again. I am six years old. I never see the car coming. The poor guy who hit me had just come back from the hospital after having had a heart attack. Running over a small child was the last thing he needed. My brother ran into the house screaming, "Mom, Mom, Marc got hit by a car!"

The next sound I heard was my mother running out of the house screaming, "Oh my God! Oh my God!" As a trained nurse, she expected the worst. I was more scared than anything, and I didn't need medical attention. The fear around that incident resulted in a new house for us down the street, in a cul-de-sac.

Even by second grade, I knew my interest in school was wavering. The always-present memory of the kindergarten spaceship fiasco fueled my defiance. "Rambunctious" and "uncontrollable" were the first multisyllabic words I learned. They were as truthful as they were descriptive. I just liked being outdoors: free to run and play to my heart's content. When I was old enough to sign up for organized sports in our community, I signed up for all of them.

Why not? Miami offers a climate that is conducive to twelve months of outdoor sports. There is no off-season. This is one reason South Florida has some of the best young athletes in the country. For me, it was all sports, all year-round. In the fall, it was football; autumn, basketball; spring, baseball, and in the summer, I went off to sleep-away camp.

I started going to sleepaway camp when I was eight. Catholic Charities sponsored Camp San Pedro. It was located in a remote area of Orlando called Goldenrod. It wasn't as if my brother and I had any choice in the matter. My parents said we were going to camp, and that was it, end of discussion. I guess they figured out that if they wanted some free time away from the kids, camp was a great solution. Unlike today when parents are overbearing and don't let children out of their sight, it was quite the opposite in the 1970s. We were encouraged to leave the house and not bother coming back until dinnertime. Camp gave my parents a few weeks off. It was a practice that continued until I went to high school.

After a couple years at San Pedro, my brother was done with camp. I was growing in independence and confidence too. I was ready for a new adventure, and a new camp called Twin Lakes offered me even more freedom.

Twin Lakes was a coed camp located a few miles outside of Boone, North Carolina. Surrounded by the Blue Ridge Mountains, Twin Lakes had an expanded variety of sports and activities. Most significantly, it also provided the novelty of girl campers. For four years, it was the place I went to get away from home. Not only did I become proficient in all the activities, including rifle shooting, horseback riding and jumping, canoeing, hiking, and all the sports, but my biggest and most impressionable experience was the introduction to the wonderment of women.

The beauty of Twin Lakes was that everybody—especially crucial, the girls—attended a different school than I in Miami. This gave me the opportunity to rebrand myself. I had a fresh start without the labels and bad reputation that I was earning at home. I had a clean slate. I served up a new image and personality to match my new setting. The girls were a different breed. They hadn't been brainwashed in the Catholic doctrines. They seemed more liberal when it came to sexual relations. Without getting into specific details, and to be able to have my three nieces read this book, let's just say that I was still a virgin when my four summers at Twin Lakes Camp terminated, but only technically.

Needless to say, I loved camp! But it was time to move on. High school was beginning and my childhood was ending. Time to become a man.

It was also a time when the wheels of growth were slowly grinding. The Miami of the 1980s and 1990s was just starting to emerge. Miami Beach was predominantly a retirement haven. Put it this way: the only real sign of life on South Beach was Joe's Stone Crab restaurant and a haunting, dilapidated building that housed a dog track. The ethnic mix that defines Miami now was slowly percolating, but it was nowhere to be found back then. The city was older, slower, and easier to navigate. Change was coming, but Miami, still more like a large town, was an easy, wonderful place to grow up.

Our new home was only six houses away from our first one. It sat on three-quarters of an acre surrounded on three sides by a canal that opened up to a large lake. Since the house was built for us, it had everything—a swimming pool, basketball court, and large backyard perfect for football. My brother and I spent countless hours in that canal, sometimes fishing for bass and bream, other times diving for turtles or just swimming.

With a tough older brother, even tougher old school Catholic nuns, and a mother who trumped them all—this, in a house with a future Hall of Fame football player—it paid to be adaptive in mind and spirit. My reflexes became keen, and my demeanor savvy, as I was often required to adjust to my circumstances in ways that would best ensure my well-being.

My mother was strict to the same degree Muhammad Ali was light on his feet. My free spirit clashed with her sense of discipline. That made our home life volatile, or at least that's how it seemed to her youngest son. Gina was on the fair side of perfect—a solid citizen, good in school, rarely in trouble, and an all-around nice person. Nicky had many of the same attributes; though "nice" was not a word I ever used to describe him. He was tough, football tough, and he was big-brother mean. He also was competitive, driven, and fearless. Nicky enjoyed nothing more than to use me as a prop to display his tough-ness, usually for nothing more than the sport of it.

Actually, I was afraid of my brother and with good reason. He is two-and-a-half years older than I and that's a big difference when you're seven or eight years old. He messed with me all the time, con-stantly pounding me into submission. A lot of the crazier things I did for the first time were the result of a simple calculation.

"Marc, jump out of the tree into the canal."

"No, man, no, I can't do it."

"If you don't do it, I'm going to kick your ass."

Out of the tree I would go.

Still, I always looked up to Nicky because he accomplished so much. When he and his friends were around, I wanted to be part of their group. I wanted to be accepted by him because I admired all those characteristics of his that were different from mine. That's just what little brothers do. No matter how much I wanted to be close to my brother, it was a combustible, and oftentimes volatile relationship. And when it came to confrontation, I was always on the receiving end. It ended up being a one-way fight just about all the time. He'd whale on me and I would either be covering up or trying to run away. I knew if he caught me it would be far worse. What kinds of things would he do? How about rubbing duck shit in my face while he held me down on the ground, or spitting on my face as he held me in place? You know, brotherly love.

My mother and father never knew anything about what my brother did to me. Why not? Simple. He scared me into silence. He told me, "If you say anything to Mom or Dad, then this is nothing. You think this is bad? Just wait to see what happens if you tell them."

I never said a word because I knew it was true. Whatever my brother did to me was going to be far worse than anything my parents might do to him.

You ever play kill the man with the ball? Nicky would have all his friends over, then pick up a football and hand it to me. Then he'd announce the game: "Let's play 'kill the man with the ball!'" Nicky would pick me up and body-slam me onto the ground. That was fun. Ironically, although I received most of the punishment growing up, it was my brother who often ended up at the hospital.

I don't know if he was accident-prone, or just clumsy. My dad is definitely clumsy, to the point that it's part of family lore. It was a miracle to get through dinner without my dad spilling a glass of wine or dropping a utensil or two on the floor. My brother had a lot of slips and falls, but not because he wasn't a great athlete. Nicky was reckless, just like me. We were playing Kick the Can one night. Nicky jumped over a hedge and caught his leg on a sprinkler head. The sprinkler ripped his leg wide open from his knee to the ankle. It took one hundred stitches to close the wound. Playing football one day in our backyard, Nicky dove over me to score a touchdown and broke his hand on the landing. Another time we were riding bikes toward a neighbor's driveway that had just been repaved. It was extra slippery due to a recent rain. Nicky hit his brakes and flew off the bike straight into a coral wall, splitting his head wide open. And that's before all the subsequent football injuries and surgeries.

I was neither clumsy nor accident-prone. When I was younger I had acute nephritis, which is inflammation of the kidneys. Kidneys secrete what is essentially a poison that has to be released from the kidney. When it's not released, it can cause serious problems. When I was about six years old, I ended up spending a week in the hospital. Then, about once a year I would get really bad headaches, like migraines. I had a lot of bloody noses too. I could sneeze or laugh just hard enough and get a bloody nose. One night a bunch of friends and I went to Howard Johnson's for ice cream. I was laughing so hard that a blood clot flew out of my nose and onto my ice cream. As my disgusted friends looked on in disbelief, I moved it to the side and kept on eating. It was a Fabulous Fudge Delight, so of course I wasn't going to let a little blood clot come between me and ice cream.

But I never broke a bone. Otherwise, I was perfectly healthy.

I was always a good athlete, and I became adept at avoiding the consequences of most hazards though I tempted fate as often as possible and had a near-absolute fearlessness. My brother and I would climb trees that were forty to fifty feet high and do one-and-a-half flips off of them into the canal. I used to do flips out of a tree onto a neighbor's trampoline. I jumped off houses. I did free dives down fifty to sixty feet underwater. We also had a little "john boat," one of those little flat aluminum boats with a five-horsepower motor on the back that we took out fishing.

One of our made-up fun inventions involved using some boards to construct a ramp. Then we tied ropes to the back of our bikes and rode them as fast as we could off the ramp into the canal, flying off just as the bike would hit the water. There were alligators in the canal but it never occurred to us, or our parents, for that matter, to worry about them. Besides, I never saw any *really* big ones.

We also antagonized the neighbors from time to time. We'd steal duck eggs and throw them at our neighbors across the canal, or shoot lizards and birds with our BB guns. If that got boring, my brother would point the gun at me and say, "Run."

"No!" I'd yell.

"The faster you run, the less it's going to hurt."

He was right.

I'd make a break for it. Within three or four steps, I'd feel the BBs hit me in the ass before falling to the ground in pain and agony. Nicky and his friends laughed hysterically.

My brother was worse than me when it came to messing with the neighbors, though I learned well. We had a neighbor who raised bees. One day we threw grapefruits at the beehives, and then jumped into the canal when the bees came flying out. You know, fun stuff for ten- or twelve-year-old kids.

But don't think for a minute that my mom let us get away with so much folly. Our house was known as the "Polish Training Camp" because my mother is part Polish. As soon as the front door opened, and it didn't matter who was coming into the house, the call went out: "Take off your shoes!" Our house was almost always spotless, with every chair, vase, and photograph perfectly positioned. To put it in even more perspective, after doing the dishes or getting a drink out of the kitchen faucet, or after brushing our teeth and using the bathroom sink, the job wasn't complete until you dried every drop of water in the sink. I used to think to myself, "Dry the sink?" But that's my mother. She is a neat freak and a devout Catholic who has a deeply held belief in the old saw that cleanliness is next to godliness. And if you wanted to question that philosophy, she would fall back to Proverbs: "He who spares the rod hates his son, but he who loves him is careful to discipline him."

My friends were scared of my mom. We were far more worried about how my mother would respond to an indiscretion compared to what my dad might do. Every once in a while, when the incident was particularly bad, we would hear, "Wait until your father gets home."

Of course, whenever anything went wrong in the neighborhood it was always the Buoniconti boys. We were immediately under suspicion. When a neighbor came to our door to complain, my mom wouldn't even argue our guilt or innocence. All she would say is, "OK, what did they do now?" A couple times the cops showed up and that was the kind of thing that would move the discipline from my mom to my dad. We didn't do anything really bad, just kid stuff.

On Halloween we threw smoke bombs into a house here and there. We'd ring the doorbell and run, or do the old garbage can trick by leaning a can filled with urine against the front door and ring the bell. Whoever opened the door would get a river of urine running into their house. That's back when kids had to be creative and invent our fun. We didn't have video games, cell phones, or computers.

When he got into high school, Nicky enjoyed going out and having a good time, but he was much more focused on school than I was. He studied hard and was an all-around leader, including membership in the Fellowship of Christian Athletes. He was always doing the right thing. Aside from having a couple cocktails and getting into a few fender benders, Nicky was a straight arrow. He was captain of this, president of that. I took a different approach. I was doing the wrong thing most of the time because it was usually more fun. I wasn't captain of anything in high school until my senior football season.

* * *

NICK JR: From the perspective of a little brother, Marc might have had a different view but we were never abusive. We gave Marc a hard time because he was that little brother you see in movies tagging along with his brother and his brother's friends.

I loved my little brother, but he was still my little brother.

Make no bones about it though. Marc was as tough as anyone. It didn't matter whether it was in practice or a game. I know this: what Marc has gone through is monumental. None of us can imagine what it's like to be him or to roll in those wheels. I'm not sure anyone else in our family could have done what Marc has done.

* * *

I was in trouble in one form or another, all the time. Nothing serious, but trouble nonetheless. Yet, there were a few times I didn't deserve the punishment I received, and no discipline, however harsh, could make me apologize. If I had to stay in my room for a week, then I did the time without complaint. I was resolute and never would say I was sorry for a crime I didn't commit. On the other hand, there were far more times I didn't get the punishment my actions probably deserved. In that sense, I was a fortunate escape artist of sorts despite inviting all manner of trouble.

Then again, it wasn't hard to run outside the lines when they were as rigidly defined as they were by my mother. We had a living room that was off limits 364 days a year. Thick, white shag carpeting covered its floor. My mother used to rake the carpet to eliminate any trace of an actual human footstep. We were only allowed into that room on Christmas. Then, twelve months later to the day, we'd be allowed back again.

Put it this way. When my father retired from the Dolphins in 1976, my mother took his trophies, awards, certificates, and all related evidence of a glorious sports career, loaded them into a box, and told my dad to take them out to the garage.

"Your football career is over now," she said. "Now it's time to be a regular husband and father."

My father wore the pants in our house, but my mother had a pair made especially for her too. She did a great job of keeping everyone grounded.

Although I turned out to be a pretty good football player, I probably was even better in the water. Whether it was scuba diving, swimming, water skiing, hydro-sliding, fishing, spearfishing, or free diving into the ocean, it all came naturally to me. Being on and in the water was my first love. I swam competitively when I was young and I was good, really good. I don't think I ever lost a race in the first six years I competed. My mother used to get embarrassed at swim meets. Every time I was awarded a blue ribbon I'd climb into the stands and give it to her. By the end of the meet she had a stack of blues and, needless to say, some of the other parents didn't think it was nearly as endearing as my mother did.

The one story she tells about my swimming exploits involved a neighbor. They lived across the street and had a son about my age. He took formal swimming lessons for years and he had all the latest gear—the Speedo swimsuit, racing goggles, everything. I never had any formal instruction. I showed up for the meets and swam in whatever shorts I happened to be wearing that day. My mother said it was like I had a motor attached to me. One summer I attended a swimming camp with the neighbor kid. When the big meet came along, I wore my usual shorts and I left him in my wake in every race. According to my mother, the kid's mom was so mad that she never spoke to her again.

My friends and I would spend every waking moment, even during the school year, fishing in the canals around our neighborhood, as well as in the local spots along the shores of Biscayne Bay.

Later on, we pushed the limits of fishing just like we did with everything else. I learned the art of free diving and spearfishing during weekend boating trips to the outer reefs of Miami and the Bahamas. Unlike scuba diving, which requires oxygen tanks, free diving is done with nothing more than a mask, snorkel, and fins. I would routinely dive fifty to sixty feet into the ocean with a spear and hold my breath for up to two to three minutes before resurfacing.

I also mastered what is called a "Hawaiian Sling," which is like a slingshot with a five-foot stainless steel spear. One of the best summers of my life was between tenth and eleventh grades when my friend Charlie Richards and I spent every day free diving the patch reefs outside of Elliott Key collecting conch and spearfishing. It wasn't unusual in a given day to shoot twenty fish—a mix of grouper, snapper, lobster, and whatever fetched the highest price—weighing up to twenty pounds apiece. We'd clean all the fish and conch and sell our haul to Captain's Tavern Seafood Market where my brother worked. Charlie and I would each make one hundred dollars per day cash; not a bad summer job for someone who loved the water as much as I did. There was a real peace and tranquility about hitting the water and diving down deep into another world.

But that much time spent in the water wasn't without risk. When you are free-diving fifty to sixty feet holding your breath, there's an adrenaline rush that comes with chasing, then spearing, a fish. It was an exhilarating feeling to be so connected to nature and entering another animal's domain. That's why I never used a spear gun. I thought it was unfair. I thought my success or failure should be based on skill and tenacity. I didn't want an advantage.

There were many times when I looked up and saw fifty feet of water above me while my lungs screamed for air. I sometimes didn't know whether I could make it to the surface, but that's how I how I lived my life. I thrived on pushing myself to the extreme, to the farthest edge.

Needless to say, it was a great time to be growing up in Miami, even better if you were associated with the Miami Dolphins. The Dolphins were the only professional sports team in the state of Florida in the 1970s and 1980s. The next closest professional sports team of any kind was nearly seven hundred miles away in Atlanta. After Atlanta, the next closest NFL team was in Washington, DC, more than a thousand miles straight north. And those Dolphins turned out to be one of the great teams in NFL history by winning the Super Bowl in back-to-back seasons while recording the league's only undefeated season.

I was only ten years old when my father retired in 1976. It wasn't until I started to play football that I fully appreciated what the

Buoniconti name meant in Miami. I played Pop Warner football starting with the seventy-five-pound team for the Kendall Broncos. No matter where we played, I'd hear kids chanting before the game, "We want Buoniconti." I used that as a motivational chant. By the end of the fourth quarter, the last thing they wanted was more Buoniconti.

Richmond Heights and the Palmetto Raiders teams were made up of all African-American kids while the Tamiami and Hialeah teams were all Hispanics. I played running back and linebacker and we always had a great team. In 1980 my Kendall Broncos team was considered one of the best Pop Warner teams ever to play in South Florida.

My parents were supportive, but they never made a big deal about the fact that my father played professional football. Not only do I never remember throwing a football around with my dad, he made a point of being a quiet observer. He coached our baseball teams and my sister's softball team, but he never made suggestions to our coaches on the football field.

The Dolphins were the kings of Miami in those days, but at our house my dad was just another husband with a job. My mother kept him grounded, that's for sure. But one thing never in doubt in our home was the love we had for one another. I was in trouble a fair amount of time, but I loved my mother and father, and I knew they loved me.

Chapter 2

The Sweet Life

MOM: Nick and I were high school sweethearts. We grew up in Springfield, Massachusetts, in the 1950s. Both of our grandparents were immigrants, so our parents were first-generation Americans. Since my father was Italian and my mother was Polish, we were considered to live in the "American" neighborhood. Everyone in Nick's neighborhood was Italian.

It was funny because Nick's mom noted that I wasn't "all Italian." But I was 100 percent Catholic and that went a long way. I sold Nick a raffle ticket in ninth grade, and he still says it's the most expensive ticket he has ever bought. We were fourteen years old at the time. He grew up in the south end, right behind the Mt. Carmel Church. Nick was an altar boy.

All of his family, which included thirteen aunts, would come over every Sunday for dinner. I couldn't tell them apart for a long time. His grandfather was sweet, and all his aunts were nice. Nick had a nice upbringing, just like I did.

My dad worked twenty-five years in circulation for the *Springfield Union* newspaper. Then he sold Ruppert Knickerbocker beer. My mother was a tough lady who worked in a factory. My parents worked hard and so did Nick's. His family owned a modest Italian bakery called Mercolino's on Columbus Avenue, which still exists today. His mom worked there too. There were a lot of houses where both parents had jobs. These weren't career jobs like today. Those people had to work. My mother worked 3 p.m. to 11 p.m. in a coil factory. And she never stopped working because she never forgot the pain of the Depression.

During the 1930s, she was the only one in her family who had a job. Her brother and parents weren't able to find work during the Depression and they struggled. She worked for Westinghouse in a huge factory in Springfield. There were a lot of factories in the area back then. She finished high school and went right to work. My mother couldn't imagine leaving her family because she was the only one making any money. She didn't marry my father until she was twenty-six, which at the time was considered old to be just getting married. When my grandfather died, my mom's mother came to live with us. She never learned English, so my brother and I grew up speaking Polish. When my grandmother died, my mother stopped speaking to us in Polish. My father never spoke Italian around the house. His mother said, "I came all the way to America and I am going to speak English." It was just the opposite in Nick's house, where everyone spoke Italian.

My mother wouldn't consider working anywhere other than the factory out of fear of being without a job. She didn't make much money, but she worked hard. And she was strict. We called it the Polish Training Camp, which eventually is how my kids referred to our home. My dad had a nice job, but my parents couldn't get married until the economic situation of their families became better established.

Nick and I had a little fight our senior year and it was over between us for a while. He finished high school and waved goodbye on his way to college. Then at Easter of our freshman year, he called and we got back together. Three years later we married right around Easter time of his senior year at Notre Dame. We were twenty-one years old. I was working as a registered nurse. I had completed a three-year program, so I had a job and a car, a little Falcon. It was nice. We were two kids growing up quickly, and we had three babies right away.

The first two, Gina and Nicky, are a year and two weeks apart. Then I had Marc. I had a three-year-old, a two-year-old, and a newborn. I wanted a fourth child, but I found out I was RH positive, which is an incompatibility in blood type. These days it's not a big deal, but back then it was an issue. My body essentially rejected the baby, and based on what was to come, things probably worked out for the best. Soon after, Nick was traded from Boston to Miami. He had just finished law school at Suffolk, going to class at night. There was one tall building in Miami when we moved there in 1969, the courthouse downtown on Flagler Street. The Biltmore hotel in Coral Gables was used as a navigational aid to boaters so they could find their way home. Miami was a much different place then.

Nick not only played professional football, but he had a job in the offseason too. I was very proud of him. Both of us were from very modest backgrounds, and we were thrilled with whatever came our way. There was one swimming pool for 150,000 people in Springfield when we were kids. In Miami, we had a swimming pool in our back yard.

Marc was still in diapers when we came to Miami. We arrived in June and he didn't turn three until September. He was a late bloomer when it came to getting out of diapers. I remember saying, "You know, Marc, they don't have diapers in Miami so what are we going to do?" He got out of diapers right away after that.

Nick would take Marc and Nicky to the Orange Bowl for walkthroughs on Saturdays before Sunday NFL games. That's what Marc loved to do. He was thrilled. The kids would run all over the Orange Bowl. They would run the steps and play all over the field. Marc would only occasionally go to the games because he was so young, but Nicky went. When we were still in Boston, I took Gina to one game. They actually played at Fenway Park in those days. She was so cute. A fan screamed and she started crying, so that was her last game. You forget that this little baby probably isn't going to like all the screaming and yelling.

As the boys grew up, the fact that their father played professional football was just part of their experience, no big deal. The Dolphins quarterback, Bob Griese, was at our house one day and the boys and their friends were so excited. Then someone said something about their father, Nick, being a Dolphins player, too, but about that they were unimpressed. One of the kids said, "Oh, that's just Nicky's dad." They didn't make the connection.

Later on, when the boys grew up and started playing football, they would have their teammates over to the house before a game to watch a video of the Dolphins' undefeated 1972 season, which is still an NFL record. They would sit in the family room and watch the video to get fired up for the game. Marc was born in 1966, so he was only six years old that season.

I was a strict mother. I would throw the kids out in the morning so they could play. When they came home for dinner, even with their friends, everyone had to wear a shirt with sleeves, no tank tops allowed. If their friends didn't have proper attire, then I provided it for them. My rules were non-negotiable and I expected them to be followed. Everyone had to be home at 6 o'clock for dinner. No excuses, no exceptions. There were two other big rules: Get good grades and don't lie. I always told them they didn't have to get all As. Just do your best.

Only one of the three, Nicky, took an Advanced Placement class in high school. I had two kids who worked hard for the good grades they received. Ironically, Marc might have been the smartest one, but he never studied. Nothing about school worked for Marc. The other two did pretty well.

One time I came home, and Nicky and Marc said, "Want a glass of wine, Mom?" I thought, "Why do I need a glass of wine at three in the afternoon?"

It turned out Marc had run into the bathroom to get away from Nicky. Marc locked the door, and Nicky put his fist through it trying to get a hold of Marc. They had their dad trying to patch the hole as I walked into the house. It was just boys being boys. I really didn't leave them alone that much because they were wild. But it was a different time. They could jump on their bikes and ride all over, all day. They would bike to the movies, to play baseball. They rode their bikes everywhere all the time. Now, I won't let my grandchildren out of my sight. Miami was so much smaller then.

The Mariel boatlift changed the atmosphere in Miami. In addition to all the great people who fled Cuba for a better life in America, Castro was said to have emptied his prisons too. There was talk at one point that the streets of Havana were safer than the streets of Miami for that reason. Then the drugs started to become a big business in Miami into the 1980s. We had a little boat and the boys would "Save the Bales" of marijuana floating in Biscayne Bay. I don't know if their dad knew about that either.

There was a community, Stiltsville, with about thirty houses built on stilts. All these kids would take their boats out, jump in the water, and have parties. It was just a different time. There were no cell phones. I would give them a dime in case they needed to call me from a pay phone.

Our kids took a private bus to school. Marc kept getting kicked off, so they made him take the public bus. But one time they wouldn't let him on that one either. So I called the school and said, "You know, Sister, it's too far for Marc to walk. And I'm not going to let him ride his bike on that road because it's too busy. You are punishing me because now I have to drive him to and from school every day."

That was grammar school!

Marc came home one day with a hibiscus flower for me. Right away I knew there was a problem. He handed me his report card: six Ds and one A, which he got in physical education. I was so mad that rather than kill him I tore the report card into tiny pieces. He started crying and I felt like crying, too, because now I had to tape the whole thing back together so I could sign it.

I asked him all the time, "Marc, how are you doing in school?" And he always said the same thing, "I'm doing great, mom." I went to every parent-teacher conference. I was always a room mother so I was in the school all the time. I had to go to Sister and ask her why she didn't tell us he was doing so poorly.

At one point, we sent Marc to a psychologist. He was lying all the time about everything, grades being one of them. From my perspective, he didn't seem to differentiate between a lie and the truth. Later on, of course, he told me it was easier to tell a lie than to tell me the truth because he knew he'd be on the other end of my wooden spoon. We gave the kids a smack. With Marc, in addition, I did what was called "campusing," which meant he couldn't leave the property. But he loved it. This went on right up through eighth grade.

By the time he went to high school, he was out of control. I took everything out of his room, and it didn't make any difference. I'd leave him in there with a pencil and a piece of a paper to do his homework. Three hours later I'd go in, and he was as content as could be. He didn't get one thing done, but he was fine. Marc could entertain himself with almost nothing. I was really stuck.

I was so frustrated because I didn't know how to deal with Marc. So we started sending him to a priest named Father Radloff, a Jungian analyst who worked with children. Eventually, I ended up seeing Father Radloff, which seemed to work out better.

Nothing worked with Marc.

Chapter 3

The Old School

DAD: My dad was a very unusual guy in some respects, but he loved his boys. The sun rose and set on our heads. He just loved us. He was a guy who had a big bark but a very small bite. He also had a very short fuse. He would blow up, then a minute later he was sorry, and you would see the soft side of him come out. He was a wonderful father.

When my dad was in his teens, he played baseball with a team from Springfield, barnstorming through the eastern part of the country. There were no formal minor leagues at the time. The team played in Maine, Vermont, and Connecticut. It was semi-pro baseball, and he was a ter-rific pitcher. Everyone I've ever talked to said my dad was one of the best athletes they had ever seen. He just never had the opportunity to pursue sports as a profession. First of all, he was young when he married my mom. Then he had to earn a living like everyone else. Trying to play base-ball was speculative at best, and you still needed a job to fall back on.

In his own way, he was a very mellow guy. But he was also a tough guy. He had to be tough. He was in a very tough business that demanded discipline and long hours. He worked for my grandfather in the family bakery. My grandfather made the bread, and my father delivered it. They were up at 4:30 or 5 o'clock in the morning and they never set foot back in the house until 6:30 or 7 o'clock at night. They worked long days. There was a lot of tough weather where we lived. My father had to navigate it every day. Like I said, my dad was a tough guy. When my grandfather decided to retire, he sold the bakery to my father. That's when he started doing the baking and the delivery. It's the worst business to be in because of all the brutal hours. My brother Peter is still in the family business.

Still, my dad never missed one of my football practices. How did I know that? He used to lean against a tree near the field. Even when practice was winding down and the sun was setting, I could see the glow of his cigarette. Then he would just leave. I'd go in, shower, and walk home.

My grandfather was born in Naples, Italy, and he was a great guy. We were very, very close. He didn't speak much English, and I didn't speak much Italian. One of my aunts lived with my grandfather next door to us in a duplex. They had every meal with us. I had the great opportunity to be around my grandfather and to really appreciate his heritage through his stories about coming from Italy.

He had to leave his wife and two daughters in Italy so he could come to America and find a job. Once he established himself, he sent for them. It was an interesting tale. He started off working in a button factory in New Jersey. Unbeknownst to him, one of his good friends with whom he had worked in the bakery business back in Italy settled in Springfield. My grandfather went to visit the man one day. They decided to join together and start a bakery.

My grandfather was prolific in his ability to propagate the faith. He had thirteen children, though only nine survived a flu epidemic. Every time my grandmother became pregnant, my grandfather would paint "Mercolino and Son" on the side of his delivery truck, which at the time was a horse and buggy. Then my grandmother would have a baby girl and my grandfather would have to repaint the side of the carriage. He did that about five times; then he decided it was fruitless. It's a good thing he came to that conclusion early because my grandmother had thirteen daughters. She never had a son. My grandfather never saw that wish fulfilled.

My parents had three boys, and I was the first. Living right next door, we were very close. When someone asks me about my childhood, I always say, "No one had a better childhood than I did." Having my grandfather on one side and my family around me every day, it was magic.

As I think back, it was so much simpler then. Growing up was very easy. I'd go to school, come home, grab my baseball mitt or my football helmet or my basketball, and off I went. No one had to worry about where I was going or whether I'd get in trouble. We grew up in a 100 percent Italian neighborhood. We walked the streets on a Sunday afternoon, and you could smell the sauce cooking on the stoves. It was one of those neighborhoods where the neighbors looked after all the children. It was just a matter of enjoying yourself at the church playground, which was right across the street from where I lived. Every parent was a parent to us. It didn't matter to which house you went to play, they always had something for you to eat and drink. It was a great time, just wonderful.

What I saw in my father is that in his own way he made so many sacrifices. He never complained about it. In the winter if it snowed and we didn't shovel the driveway, I'd hear my father's truck pull in, then the next thing I'd hear was the shovel. This is 6:30 at night, usually in the dark, after working thirteen or fourteen hours. So what did we do? We put on our boots, grabbed a shovel, and helped him shovel the driveway. My father was disciplined. Anybody who does what he did for so many years had to be.

He did whatever it took, which is something he probably learned growing up on a large farm he worked with his father. When my dad started dating my mother and needed a few more bucks, he started driving a truck for a food distributor. Eventually my grandfather gave him a job working in the bakery and the opportunity to move into the duplex.

I knew what hard work looked like. I saw my father do it every day. I would help him deliver bread on Saturdays. After a while he didn't want to climb up and down the steps to the second and third floors to deliver one loaf of bread. Other times, we'd be driving down the street, and I'll never forget it because it happened many, many times. He'd see a homeless man, stop the truck, and tell me to give the man a loaf of bread. There was an old black guy who my father would see once every two weeks. He would stop the truck and tell me, "Give him a loaf of bread." The man came up to the truck one day and said, "God bless you, sir. Thank you so much." I've never forgotten that. As tough as my father was, he was really a mush. I guess that's who I am too. I can't stand seeing animals mistreated. I won't step on an ant. I can't kill anything. That's why I've never been able to hunt. I don't even like to fish because I actually don't want to catch one. I like to eat seafood as long as someone else catches it. I'm really a Buddhist at heart. I could live a Buddhist life, which certainly isn't how I was brought up. We were good Catholics. I went to Catholic school all the way through college.

I attended Notre Dame, but it wasn't a choice I would have made by myself. I wanted to stay close to Springfield. I had such close relationships with my friends and my family. I didn't want to go outside the state. I applied to Harvard, Holy Cross, Boston College, Amherst, Williams, and Yale. At the time, Holy Cross had a good football team, and all those schools recruited me. What kind of tipped the scales was a trip my father and I took to South Bend. When my father saw the Golden Dome on Notre Dame's campus, he was just so enamored of it that he couldn't imagine me going anywhere else. I wasn't nearly as enamored of it as he was.

I was getting letters from a lot of different schools from all over the country. Even Al Davis, the Oakland Raiders owner, was trying to recruit me to the University of Southern California. He was kind of like the director of player personnel at USC at the time. I was getting five or six letters a week from different schools that wanted me to come out for a visit. Now, I was only 5-feet-11 and 190 pounds. I wasn't a big guy, but I had some very good years in high school. I would take the letters down to my high school coach, Billy Wise. He helped me probably more than anybody other than my dad. He was a major influence in my life. We'd sit there and sort through the letters. He would tell me about each school, which ones were solid academically, which ones were just football factories.

Then all of a sudden, the letters stopped. I went to the principal's office to see Sister Mary Eugene. I said, "Sister, I don't know what happened. I was getting letters every week and all of a sudden, they stopped. Do you have them here?"

She looked at me and said, "Didn't you get a solicitation from Notre Dame?"

I told her I had.

"Did you fill out the application?"

"Yes," I responded.

"Isn't Notre Dame a Catholic school?"

"Yes it is, Sister."

"Well, I've been throwing all the rest of them away."

Between her and my father it was a foregone conclusion. There were a couple guys from Springfield who preceded me at Notre Dame. One of them was Angelo Bertelli, the Heisman Trophy winner. Angelo went to my high school, so he was an influence on me. Another guy, Milt Piepul, was an All-American at Notre Dame, and at the same time Joe Scibelli, who was from Springfield and went on to play for the Rams for thirteen years, was at Notre Dame doing great. So there were a lot of influences.

My greatest attributes were quickness and instinct. I was able to read what was unfolding and get to the play. It's sort of like a great running back. You can't teach a fast runner how to see the hole. Great running backs instinctively know where to go. They turn a small hole into a big hole. They get through it by reacting to what's happening around them. Linebackers are the same way because there are a lot of things going on in any given play. There is so much movement at the line of scrimmage, yet you have to observe it, analyze it, and commit.

I had a good time at Notre Dame, and I played a lot. My senior year, I started on both sides of the ball, which a lot of guys did back then. I led the team in tackles as a linebacker and it looked like I had a good chance to play in the National Football League.

Terry was my high school sweetheart. We were married April 28, 1962. We married in April for one reason—to save money. She had planned to come to Notre Dame for my senior prom and my graduation. I said, "This is crazy. Why don't we get married in April? You'll already be out here, and you won't have to fly or drive back again." The original plan was to be married in June, so why not move it up and save a few bucks? Our daughter, Gina, was born eleven months later.

There were twenty rounds in the National Football League Draft when I came out of Notre Dame in 1962. The American Football League had thirty-four rounds. The draft went on for days, but there wasn't anything like ESPN making a big deal about it hour after hour like now. What shocked me was that the Chicago Sun-Times had a photograph on the back cover of the sports section leading up to the draft. It was a photograph of three players who were expected to be selected early in the draft—Bob Ferguson, a quarterback from Ohio State was picked fifth, Roman Gabriel, a quarterback from North Carolina State, who ended up being the No. 2 pick, and Nick Buoniconti from Notre Dame. I was never even selected by the NFL, not even in the twentieth round.

Eventually I found out why that happened. My college coach, Joe Kuharich, who ended up being one of the worst coaches in Notre Dame history, when asked about me by NFL teams replied, "Here's the deal. If you ask Nick Buoniconti to run through a brick wall, he'll run through a brick wall. But the hole he leaves will be small."

That was the recommendation he made to the pros. So I was considered too small. The Boston Patriots drafted me in the thirteenth round of the American Football League draft. Calgary had my rights in the Canadian Football League. When I attended the end-of-the-year football banquet at Notre Dame, the Calgary scout was there. He offered me $10,000 with a $2,000 bonus. I asked him where Calgary was. The scout said, "You know Canada? Well, we're at the far west end of Canada." I'm thinking to myself, "Well, it's either going two thousand miles to Calgary or ninety miles from Springfield to Boston. I think it's going to be the Patriots." I figured my family could come watch me every weekend. It was an easy decision, really. If I wanted to play pro ball, I really had one choice. That choice came with a $10,000 contract and a $1,000 signing bonus.

The transition was pretty seamless for me, though I was totally naïve as a rookie. Our first game of the 1962 season was against the Dallas Texans, who later moved to Kansas City and became the Chiefs. The Texans played in the Cotton Bowl. We opened up there, and I was playing only on special teams. Harry Jacobs was our starting middle linebacker. Lenny Dawson and the Dallas offense put 44 points on the board against us. Harry had a tough game, but it wasn't his fault. Dallas had a great offense that was far superior to our defense.

The following Monday we were watching game film. My head coach called me over and said, "By the way, you're starting." I started the next, and I never left the lineup from that day forward. That's how I became a starting middle linebacker in professional football, and I always thank Lenny Dawson, who many years later became my partner on our HBO show *Inside the NFL*.

Football was instinctive for me. I didn't have to think. Games were the easiest part. Coaches would tell us what to expect, but I had my own thoughts after watching game films. I'd create my own game plans based on what I saw. I always looked for keys. Inevitably, somebody did something that gave you a key as to whether the play was going to be a run or a pass. I prepared. That's how I was able to be in the right place at the right time

Someone sent me an article that quoted my coach, Mike Holovak. He said, "Nick Buoniconti is the best middle linebacker in the AFL." This was right after my rookie year.

My first offseason I worked selling insurance, which I hated. I made a couple hundred bucks a week. But I found myself wondering where I was going with that job. If I got hurt playing football, I didn't have anything to fall back on.

I realized back then that football was never going to be able to provide me with enough money to live the kind of lifestyle I saw for my family. That's when I started going to law school at night. It was such a grind, I can't tell you. Not to pat myself on the back, but looking back, I can't imagine how I did it. I was practicing professional football during the day. Then I'd have lunch with some of the guys on the team and about 3 o'clock I'd head to the law library to study. I'd study Monday, Wednesday, and Friday from 3 o'clock to 6 p.m. I'd brief some cases, prepare for the classes, and then attend class from 6 p.m. to 9 p.m. When classes were over, I'd drive forty minutes back home and eat dinner around 10 o'clock at night. Then the next morning I'd get up, go to practice, and do it all over again. I went to class three days a week and the other days I went to the law library after practice.

It was no easier in the offseason. I had a job with the Polaroid Corporation in human resources. At night, I went to law school. It was a real grind. We had three children quickly, and they were looking for their daddy too. I can still picture them. When I wasn't away playing football, I'd come home from work or school, and their noses would be pressed up against the glass door waiting for me. It was great.

All three kids were born in Massachusetts. Terry was so understanding. She knew that my going to law school and being gone all the time meant a lot to our future. But we had three kids in diapers. We made it work because that's what you do when you have a family. We would take turns feeding, changing diapers, and waking up at night to take care of one of them. Back then it was just what you did. Now everything is a burden, an encumbrance. Not us. We understood that it was life, our life. There was no need to complain about it.

During football season, when everybody was going to play golf or head to the beach after practice, I had my law books with me. Every year the team went on a three-week road trip that took us from Boston to Denver, San Diego, and Oakland. I'd be gone about sixteen days because in those days you didn't fly back across the country after the games until the road trip ended.

I'd have to call one of my buddies in class to find out which cases had to be briefed. I had to keep up with my reading, too, without getting class-room instruction for almost three weeks. When the trip was finally over, I'd go to my professors. They would take the time to sit down with me and go through a lot of what I missed. That's why I established a scholarship at Suffolk University Law School. It was a great experience for me under the circumstances. It was a unique way to get your law degree, but I would never recommend it to anyone.

It's like anything else. Once I make my mind up to do something, I do it. It doesn't matter what it is. When I was traded from Boston to Miami in 1969, I was determined to get a guaranteed contract. I was not going to move my wife and three children from Boston, where I had just passed the Massachusetts bar and established a law practice with two young guys, without a guarantee. I was working in the district attorney's office at the time getting my feet wet prosecuting cases. I knew I had a good future as an attorney if I just stayed in Boston.

I demanded a three-year guaranteed contract. I was at the height of my career. If I played, then I had to play for Miami because the Dolphins traded for my rights. But I didn't have to play. No one could make me play. I had the leverage. They needed someone like me on the team but there were no guaranteed contracts at the time. What I was asking for was unprecedented. Joe Robbie, the Dolphins owner, refused to give me a guaranteed contract, so I said, "Fine."

I sent a letter of resignation to the league office. I retired from football. I was in the district attorney's office every day that summer. I continued to work out every day, too, but I felt that if Miami wouldn't give me a guar-anteed contract, then they would trade my rights to another team that might. I thought I might end up playing somewhere, but I had planned for my life without football.

In the final analysis, football camp was about ready to start and Joe Robbie's general manager, Joe Thomas, called me. He said, "Mr. Robbie would like you to come down to Miami and talk." Joe Thomas had a great eye for talent, and he was a very good general manager.

"Joe, if Mr. Robbie isn't going to give me the guaranteed contract, then why should I bother flying to Miami?"

"Why don't you just fly down? You never know what is going to happen."

I flew to Miami and the three of us had dinner that night. We finished dinner and Joe Robbie had a little too much to drink, so Joe Thomas and I basically carried him to bed. I went back to my room, went to sleep, and scheduled a wake-up call at 7 a.m. so I could make the 9:30 a.m. flight back to Boston.

At 7:30 a.m. I received a call from Joe Thomas. He said Mr. Robbie wanted to have breakfast. I said, "Look, I'm not going to go through this charade again." Joe insisted, so I went downstairs to have breakfast. Midway through the breakfast, Joe Robbie put his hand out across the table and said, "You have your deal, a three-year guaranteed contract."

I think the numbers were $35,000, $42,000, and $47,000. That meant I had to un-retire, which at the time was not such an easy thing to do.

My philosophy is very simple. I remember a quote that has always stuck with me: Perseverance wins success. That's how I live my life. If you persevere long and hard enough, then somehow, someway you will have at least a modicum of success. Most people aren't willing to put in the work.

Chapter 4

Fingernails on the Chalkboard

Our family went to Mass every Sunday. I attended Catholic schools from first grade all the way through high school. Still, I was what could be described as "disruptive" in school; nothing mean-spirited or hurtful to anyone in particular. I was just a kid having fun, which happened to be a foreign concept to the nuns and brothers who attempted to educate me.

I'm talking about old-school nuns at Epiphany, the grade school I attended for eight years starting in first grade. In addition, their traditional conceptions of education involved rote memorization and mechanical teaching methods, and some of them were just flat-out mean. Pulling a kid's hair, slapping somebody, or slamming a ruler across a kid's head or hands? Those were common everyday occurrences.

With the exception of first grade, I hated elementary school. It was just so boring to me. Almost nothing about school interested me. I felt even then that it was a stupid waste of time. What did I struggle with most? Everything. I was a poor student from the beginning. The idea of "Attention Deficit Disorder" wasn't a hot topic at the time. Back then you moved through the ranks, grade-to-grade, year-to-year, with the ever-present expectation of being whacked by your parents and teachers on account of poor grades. There were no qualms about using whatever means necessary to keep kids in line, and apparently to help us learn. My mom was no different. Now, I admit that I deserved just about every bit of it. Still, I was just a kid.

With that said, it's also true that I challenged everyone and everything throughout my entire school experience. I earned my first F in third grade. If I was sent to my room to study, I'd spend hours drawing pictures or making a cardboard basketball hoop and shooting baskets with wads of paper. Or I'd stare into the ceiling and count the cracks. I'd do anything but study.

What bothered me most about my Catholic education was what seemed to me the use of brainwashing as a form of discipline. There wasn't a day that went by that I didn't question the idea that God was an all-loving figure beyond our imagination. I was reminded at just about the same time that I was having some form of earthly judgment and punishment exacted on me. The nuns told us to behave or God wouldn't love us, or that we wouldn't be allowed into heaven because of our behavior. That is terrible. We were kids goofing around. We weren't getting into heaven? What kind of lesson was that?

One could argue that a teacher is justified in certain circumstances of going to just about any length to preserve order in a classroom full of noisy, misbehaving kids. Again, I don't entirely disagree. Controlling a classroom can be a daunting task for anyone. Although discipline was not a novel concept to me in any regard, what made me skeptical about the Catholic approach was the glaring hypocrisy. How could a nun, who dedicated her life to the selfless acts of Jesus Christ, treat God's children that way?

From my vantage point, they wore the habit and said the prayers, but when it came to the most important part, forgiveness, the concept escaped them. I experienced daily contradictions between what we read in the Bible and what we were living day-to-day. One thing is for sure: The experience made an indelible impression on me—as it did on many I grew up with. It drove us away from Catholic formalities.

When I was in seventh grade and preparing for Confirmation, my buddy Pat Sheehy and I were caught talking in church by Sister Jeanne. There was a large banner at the front of the church with the name of every kid about to be confirmed. Just for talking, she took our names off the banner and threw us out of the church. She took us outside and said, "You don't deserve the Holy Spirit. You're not going to get confirmed with your class." This happened early in the week leading up to the Sunday of Confirmation. Pat and I were the only ones in the class whose names weren't on the banner. The stress and anxiety that I experienced through that entire week was overwhelming. I had no idea whether or not I was going to be confirmed. Of course, I didn't say a word to my parents. As far as they knew everything was fine. When I walked into the church on the day of Confirmation I still didn't know. My brother and sister were my sponsors. By the grace of God, I was confirmed without a hitch. Apparently, not even a nun could come between me and the Holy Spirit. I still don't think there is anything educationally effective about that whole experience. She was just plain mean. For what? Talking in church. That nun is around to this day.

I received punishment from all ends and for every reason imaginable, often landing me in my room, alone with my thoughts. But I always said to myself, "If you can't enjoy your own company, then whose company can you enjoy?" I could entertain myself. My mother would "campus" me to the yard and sometimes even to my room. That meant I couldn't leave the premises—a kind of house arrest. It never bothered me, though. If I had to stay in the yard, I'd fish, shoot baskets, or hit a tennis ball against the garage door. I had no problem spending an entire day alone entertaining myself. I could be perfectly content even sitting around watching the sunset. As a kid, I loved to relax. I never had a problem finding a way to pass the time.

I did my own thing not in spite of anybody and not for any particular reason. I wasn't rebellious simply to be rebellious. I went about life according to whatever I wanted to do at the moment. I never spent much time worrying about what anyone else thought. I just didn't conform. As a result, school was always a source of trouble. It was a constant stress on my life, to say the least. My mother tried to help by arranging tutors, special classes at a learning center, and dishing out enough punishment to flip a felon.

Then there were the nuns who also had no problem dishing out punishments, whether in the form of detentions, or physical and even psychological abuse. Not to mention, my reputation got around. In the minds of other teachers, I became known not only as a bad student but as a bad kid too. My defense? I liked to have fun. It was really nothing more than that. Part of the problem was the company I kept. I met Scott "Dodie" DeNight in first grade in 1972. Everyone called him "Rodent" for the longest time, a name given to him by his brothers. Scott was the fourth of five boys. He learned plenty from the older ones, who were every bit as wild as our group. His father, Bill, a tough Irish businessman, and his mother, Sylvia, an Italian no taller than five feet, always made their presence known. Another friend, Scott "Weasel" Bistrong, the oldest of seven, came to Epiphany in fourth grade. We all loved the same things inside and outside of school.

For example, we loved to fish. We woke up at 5 a.m. on Saturdays, jumped on our bikes, and rode ten miles to our favorite fishing spot. How many ten- to twelve-year-olds do that nowadays? We were gone the entire day, fishing the whole time.

I spent a lot of time at Dodie's house, a few blocks away from mine. His house provided me safe refuge from the trouble and turmoil that was commonplace at my house. You could never be completely relaxed at my house because you never knew when something or someone was going to blow up. It was like being on constant alert. It was my mom who gave the orders. Every weekend I did my best to find a place to sleep over away from my house. If it wasn't Dodie's or Weasel's house, then you could find me just about every weekend at Pat Sheehy's house. Pat's parents, Tom and Connie, were much more liberal than my parents. As soon as I was dropped off at their house, I felt the release of stress and tension that had been building during the week.

Pat's dad was a pilot for Delta Airlines. He had the cushiest job because he was never "at work." Unlike my father, who only coached my Little League baseball team for two years, Tom coached every sport, every year, including our 1980 115-pound Pop Warner championship football team. Tom also had a lot of awesome hobbies, all of which involved high-speed and adrenaline. He raced Unlimited hydroplane boats. He drove for some of the top teams, including the Miss Madison, the Natural Light, and the Irish Mist. Pat and I would go to the annual hydroplane races on Key Biscayne at the Miami Marine Stadium. Tom also drove race cars up and down the Florida coast in the International Motor Sports Association. And when he wasn't doing either of those, he was showing off in his 911 Porsche Carrera, or his totally tricked out, customized van, loaded with all the bells and whistles including mag wheels, side exhaust pipes, refrigerator, plush carpet, and a couch that turned into a bed. It goes without saying that hanging out with the Sheehys was certainly more enjoyable than hanging at my house.

In school, we would dare one another to do something that in our minds added some fun to the day. After a test we'd compare our awful grades and try to make light of the situation, which isn't easy to do when you score 37 on a 100-point scale. I didn't care for school, but I never felt good about disappointing my parents or getting poor grades. Ultimately, I had to bring home a report card that my parents had to sign. As you can imagine, nothing was more stressful for me than report card day.

One day I received my report card and was heading home. When it came time to get off the bus, my friend Chris Doane, who lived on my street, asked, "Hey Marc, do you want to hang out later?"

"Dude, it's report card day. What are you talking about? You aren't going to see me for a month."

I wasn't consciously trying to screw up, really. I just didn't do well in school and neither did many of my friends. It wasn't like I spent any less time at home than other kids did; I had to be home by 6 o'clock every night for dinner. That was mandatory in our house. I couldn't go out all night on the weekends. I cared about school. I just didn't care enough about it to jeopardize all those things that would provide adventure and fun. Everyone has to make sacrifices in life; unfortunately, I chose to sacrifice school. Although I could handle being in my room, that doesn't mean there weren't were plenty of times I sat in my room angry and upset because I didn't do well on a test or because my report card sucked. It all just made me hate school even more.

Another source of anxiety was the fact that my brother and sister both worked really hard and did well. They were consistently recognized as first or second honors, earning As and Bs. "Why can't you be more like your brother and sister?" I heard that a hundred times. Eventually, my parents sent me to a specialist. They were concerned that I might have a learning disability. It turned out that I did. The screeners said I was one of the first documented ADHD cases they had seen. That was just as Ritalin was coming out, but I never took any medication.

When the tests came back confirming a learning disability, my parents were more bothered by the results than I was. Here is my mom for you. She apologized, telling me, "I'm sorry for punishing you, or yelling at you about school. I didn't realize you had a real problem. I am so sorry."

That lasted about three days. Then it was back to, "Try harder! You're using this learning issue as a crutch."

From the very beginning I was terrible in math, but I was creative. In our society, we deemphasize the classes that require creativity and imagination—those places where kids like me could fully express themselves. Instead, we hire more tutors. I was up to my elbows in tutors. I suppose it makes sense to one degree or another, except all this happens at the expense of developing the child's true talents and passions. So what happens? A kid like me ends up hating school.

Maybe I should have been an architect, which of course would have required math. I loved to draw. I would draw houses on my own time, away from school. I'd sketch the inside of the house and create every aspect of it. The classes I did enjoy had a visual element to them, such as history and geography, where maps were utilized. All of this was lost in a linearly defined system. Potential was summarily dismissed if it didn't line up with the pedagogy of that time.

I guess you could say I just never really got with the program.

Chapter 5

Two Wild Boys and a Girl

GINA: I am three and a half years older than Marc and a year older than Nicky. To say the least, our house was wild when we were children. My mother was extremely strict, but she had to be because we were so wild. We had a lot of freedom that was typical of the times. It wasn't like today where kids have everything controlled and planned. We had very little planned. Every day was a new adventure and no one approached the day with more abandon than my brothers. We woke up in the morning and headed out into the world. If we came back at all during the day, it was only long enough to grab something to eat or drink.

There was one unbreakable big rule in our house. Everyone had to be home by 6 p.m. for dinner. Whatever you did during the hours away from home was your own business as long as you showed up relatively clean and presentable for dinner. Our parents trusted us, and they trusted the rest of society in a way that has been lost on children today. We were free to find our fun whether it was in the neighborhood or beyond.

My father's celebrity was always just there. He was playing for the Boston Patriots in the American Football League when I was born. As a girl, that part of our family life was different for me. Marc and Nicky would go to the practices; they attended summer training camp, and both of them loved being around their father and the other players. I remember going to the Saturday walkthrough with my dad in his green Eldorado Cadillac convertible. I was mortified to be in that car, but it was a cool experience. For the boys, I'm sure it all seemed like an extension of our family. For me—not so much. On game days, I'd sleep at my best friend's house. I just wasn't as interested in football as my brothers.

Most of the time, Nicky and Marc were just roaming the neighborhood. They threw tomatoes and eggs at cars. My mother wasn't the kind of person who would immediately protest in the face of a complaint about one of her children. Instead of reflexively defending her kids when someone knocked at the front door, she'd say, "What did they do now?" Some parents might open the door and immediately announce, "My son would never do that." Not my mom. She knew they were capable of just about anything.

She was strict, trust me. The house was always immaculate despite the presence of three kids running all over the place because she demanded it be that way. On Saturdays, we had to clean—vacuum, dust, make our beds, and pick up everything before we even thought of leaving the house. My friends would make fun of us because no one could leave on Saturday until my mother waved the wand.

Marc was a maniac. He had no fear, ever, of anything. He still has no fear. Our friends, the Steins, had a trampoline. Marc was a little fireball. He was small, not skinny, but strong and agile. He would climb the tree above the trampoline and do a flip down from the tree onto the trampoline. No training, nothing but an idea that he figured would be exciting. There are probably hundreds of things Marc did that could have resulted in severe injury at the least.

He would do flips at the beach like a guy who had taken years of gymnastics. He was a natural athlete with incredible agility. Everyone knows what he could do on a football field, but Marc was an amazing swimmer too.

Nicky and Marc were always in the canal behind our house. Our parents never gave it a second thought though Mike Martin, a good friend, almost died in the canal. My brother stole a huge piece of Visqueen plastic sheeting that we used as a slip-and-slide. Eventually it became dirty, so everyone jumped into the canal with it. Mike got wrapped inside and nearly drowned. Given everything that Nicky and Marc did in and out of the canal, it's amazing someone didn't get seriously hurt along the way. There were alligators in that canal, but I never saw one.

Marc was prone to ear infections, but that never stopped him from diving into the canal or driving his bike off a makeshift ramp into the water. Marc and Nicky would blow up lizards, shoot ducks with BB guns, throw duck eggs at the neighbor's house. They threw rocks at the kids across the canal from behind beautiful holly bushes that hung over our backyard into the canal. Marc could spend the entire day entertaining himself with a couple of ropes and whatever else he came up with. He was very inventive as were all the kids in those days. We had to be. My mom would throw us out of the house from morning to night. "It's a beautiful day," she'd say. "Get outside."

Everyone, even our friends, paid attention to our mother for one reason. We were afraid of her, not dad. My dad was gone a lot either traveling to play games, practicing, or in the offseason with his law practice. When he came home, he didn't want to deal with whatever we had done wrong. He wanted peace in the house. That wasn't always easy with Marc because he truly had no fear of anything or anyone. He never really respected authority of any kind whether it came from our parents or the Catholic church. Ever.

My dad would plead with Marc, "Come on Marc, play the game. Just play the game. When your mom says something, just do it. If she wants you to apologize, just say you're sorry. Come on, Marc, it's simple."

Marc didn't care. If Mom got mad at him and Marc didn't believe he was wrong, there was no chance he would apologize no matter how harsh the punishment. He spent a lot of time alone in his room, but he never wavered. He had his own code. If he didn't believe he had committed a crime, then he couldn't be broken.

* * *

NICK JR: I probably didn't appreciate the extent of all the things going on with Marc. He was just my little brother. I chalked it up to immaturity. He probably wasn't that far off the average. But in our house, there was more emphasis on grades, toeing the line, making the right choices, and working hard. Still, I wasn't concerned about him.

Make no bones about it. While Marc did have that kind of free life-style, he was as intense and as tough as anyone. It didn't matter if it was practice or games. He had the same attributes as everyone in our house growing up.

Chapter 6

My Son Is Howard Roark

DAD: Marc was basically trouble though he was a phenomenal athlete. My son Nicky was the most determined. Once he started playing, it was not a matter of would a job get done, but only a matter of how good of a job he would do. He was committed. He was tough. Nicky was amazing. You never had to worry about him. You put him on any field in any sport and whatever ability he had, you knew he was going to max out that ability with effort and drive.

Marc, on the other hand, was like novelist Ayn Rand's character Howard Roark. He followed his own agenda. He would get the job done with the least effort required. If it took 20 percent, then Marc would do 20 percent. If it took 40 percent, he'd do 40 percent. If it took 100 percent, then Marc gave his all to get it done. With Marc, there was always something better going on. If there was something he'd rather do, then Marc would make every effort to do it. If he could skip practice and go fishing, that's what Marc was likely to do. He was just totally the opposite of Nicky.

Marc had my natural ability. He was quick like me. He had a great nose for the ball. He was just a headhunter on defense. Marc was great in coverage because he was fast enough to cover just about anybody. He played tailback and linebacker, so he had a good sense of both sides of the ball. He was just a gifted athlete.

But he was never committed to anything. He never committed to school, never committed to sports. He loved to play them as long as it suited his interest at the time. One year he came to me and said, "You know Dad, I really don't want to play football this year." This was the third or fourth week of the season. He was eight or nine at the time.

I said, "That's fine. You have to go tell your coach and teammates that you are leaving the team. But I have to tell you one thing. I don't agree with this because once you start something you should finish it. And I really don't agree with what you are doing because I believe you are letting everyone down. You are letting your teammates down, you are letting your coach down, and you are letting yourself down."

He quit.

The next year he came back to me and said, "Dad, I really want to play football this year." I said, "Here's the deal. I'll let you play, but there's no quitting. Once you start, you have to finish."

That is Marc. He is a very independent young man. Marc does what Marc wants to do. He doesn't think about the consequences. For example, he was on a team that was regarded as the best Pop Warner team in the country. He had kids on his team who were some of the best athletes I have ever seen. They were beating teams 45-0. They were just that good. The deal I had with Marc was that, if he didn't have a C average, he couldn't play. Leading up to the state championship game, he brought home a report card. I told him I wanted to see it. The championship game was a couple days away. He handed me the report card, which had magically become so stained by mud and running ink that I could hardly make out the grades. I had to call the school to find out what the card actually said. He had six Ds.

"Marc, you know what this means, don't you? You're not playing in the state championship game on Saturday." He looked at me like I was kidding. I'm sure he thought I would relent and let him play. I said, "You are going to have to go to practice and tell your coach and your teammates that, not only aren't you going to play in the state championship game, but you won't even be going to the game."

He was really ticked off at me. He went to practice and told the coach and his teammates that he couldn't play. Then I started getting phone calls from parents. They told me that I was punishing the team. I was nice about it, but I told them, "I make the rules for my own children. You aren't going to tell me what to do with my kids." So Marc didn't play, and they lost a close game, something like 14-12. Marc would have made a huge difference. Not only was he great on defense, he was a great running back on offense.

To this day Marc says, "You know, Dad, you punished me by not letting me go to that game. It didn't make any difference in my life. It didn't change me at all. You should have let me play."

"Marc, you and I had an agreement. We had a contract. You broke the contract. That's all it meant to me. I didn't care about the game."

It didn't affect him at all. In fact, he says he didn't learn a thing.

Marc was the most punished young adult ever in the history of the world. His mother used to ground him not only to the yard, but he was often confined to the house. He was always in trouble. When I was working at U.S. Tobacco in Connecticut, they sent smokeless tobacco to the house in a package. He ended up taking a couple tins on the school bus, then he handed out the chewing tobacco to kids on their way to grammar school. The bus authorities called to tell me my eighth-grade son no longer could ride the school bus in the morning. I still had a football reputation at the time, so I was able to talk them into allowing him to come back on the bus with probation.

But he was just totally intractable. Once his mother punished Marc by grounding him to his room for one week. Not in the house. I mean one week in his room. All he could do in there was study and sleep, or at least that's what he was expected to do. Well, he didn't study.

Marc never would say, "Mom, it's my fault. I'm sorry." Never. He would sit in his room and take the punishment. I'd tell him, "Marc, all you have to do is say you are sorry to your mom. Most likely she'll lift the punishment." He wouldn't do it. I would negotiate with Terry, trying to get two weeks down to one week. Every once in a while I'd say, "Marc, if you want to go on this fishing trip, then you better clear this up with your mom because, if you don't clear it up, then you're going to end up staying home with her while the rest of us go down to our house in the Keys and fish."

He would give in, but only if it suited his interests. It wasn't because he felt any compassion, remorse, or guilt. He did what Marc wanted to do at the time. It was that simple. His mother would clean out his room.

Pretty much anything that could be a distraction was removed. Marc could entertain himself doing anything, lying on his bed counting how many imperfections there were in the ceiling. He would entertain himself and never complain.

Marc never was mean. His personality was pretty docile. He didn't have an edge to him. All of my kids were much more under control than I was. I had more of my father's temperament, though kids do take on traits of the parents. For example, my daughter Gina is a lot like Terry in terms of being very disciplined and believing that cleanliness is next to godliness. Her kids come first, and everything is lined up weeks at a time. Schedules are created to be followed.

Marc is totally the opposite. Schedules exist to be changed. Appointments are made to be missed.

Chapter 7

Christopher Columbus

One day my dad called all of us into the family room. We had a nice sectional couch with a faux Chinese table. A thirty-inch television that was as big as a refrigerator had a VCR the size of a microwave sitting on top, and everything sat on an oriental rug. To one side of the room was a bumper pool table.

He announced: "Look, I've been offered a job as vice president at U.S. Tobacco, but it requires that we move to Greenwich, Connecticut. I'm going to let it be a family vote. Whatever we decide as a family will determine whether or not I take the job."

You have to remember, my dad never made a big deal about being a professional football player. It was all about family. Both of my parents made sure we understood the importance of family. We had a pretty normal life. It wasn't like he was away all the time. So when he sat us down to talk about the business opportunity we all knew he would follow the vote, one way or another.

He went on: "There is a significant salary increase. We get a very nice house and a new Cadillac Seville. We'd be living in Greenwich, which has great schools."

I don't remember anyone asking any questions. At one point, though, my sister said, "I knew it. I knew there was something going on. Oh my God. I knew it."

Once my father finished, he asked, "What do you want to do?"

Each of us cast our vote. I was ready to go, not only because it would free me from the nuns, though that was certainly part of it. I knew it was a great opportunity for my dad. I didn't mind the idea of driving around in a brand-new Cadillac Seville either. Even then I appreciated the finer things in life. I knew what they were too. We were probably upper middle class, but I aspired up the food chain. I liked nice things. I appreciated them.

I was ready to go. Why? It just so happened the timing coincided with my report card. I figured it was a good way to escape the coming storm. My logic was straightforward: let me get out of town, man, before another dose of bad news comes my way. I loved growing up in Miami, but I had enough anxiety about the coming report card to give it all up and move to Connecticut. That should put my school experience, particularly at Epiphany, in better perspective. Keep in mind I was playing football and doing really well. I was heading into eighth grade, the final hurdle before I could escape to high school. I had an established social life, and still I would have gone.

When the votes came in only two of us wanted to go – my dad and me. The others voted resoundingly "no," and that was it. We stayed.

A year later, the world changed, for me anyway. I left Epiphany and headed to Christopher Columbus High School. It was still a private Catholic environment, but I was preceded by Nicky, who had established himself as a great student and kiss ass. Actually, he was a good kid who worked hard to get good grades. And for some reason they thought I'd be the same. From my perspective, high school presented a clean slate and a breath of fresh air after eight years of hell-on-earth in grade school.

After all my trouble with grades and school in general at Epiphany, my dad gave me a pep talk before I checked into Columbus.

"Look, whatever you did in the past is over," he said. "It's important to start fresh and do well because high school is what counts when you go to college."

The Marist Brothers' approach to discipline wasn't much different than the nuns' except it was harsher, probably because Columbus was an all-boys school. My mother told the nuns, "He gets out of line, it's OK to whack him." She took the same position at Columbus until it required a slight modification: "Whack him, just not in the head." This was after I came home from school one day during my freshman year with a concussion. While this sounds extreme, you have to remember that this was typical behavior in that era.

My history teacher was a good guy, and we got along great, but he was crazy. He was the quarterback coach and offensive coordinator on the football team.

Screwing around to the point that a teacher whacked you was commonplace and often the highlight of the day. This particular teacher walked around class with what were essentially weapons. He had a large samurai sword made of wood. As if that didn't hurt enough, he also had a horsewhip with a large handle. When he cracked me with the handle of that whip, I wished he had whipped me instead. The handle was made of metal, and it was cement-hard. I never saw it coming. All of a sudden, whack, right across the back of my head. I went down to the floor. I wasn't knocked out, but I was dazed. The next day I couldn't even put my helmet on in practice because it hurt so badly. That's when my mom went to the school and said, "I don't care if you hit him, just don't hit him on the head. He's having a hard enough time at school already."

My friend Dodie and I were fooling around in this teacher's class one day when, out of nowhere, came the sword. Dodie wasn't ten feet away when the teacher fired the sword at him. The only thing that saved Dodie was that he had the presence of mind to pick up a book to block its trajectory. If he hadn't grabbed the book, the sword would have hit him square in the face. I'm not sure I would have thought to lift up the book. I was shocked. Another friend, John "Fatty" McConnon, got hit all the time just because he was a bad student. It got so bad for Fatty that he had to change schools after our head football coach took his and Dodie's heads and slammed them together for talking in church.

Chris Doane sat in the front row of our history class. He was a brilliant student and ended up becoming an electrical engineer for

General Electric. For some reason, our history teacher, the guy with the weapons, referred to Chris as "the weatherman." If it rained, the teacher would knock him around.

"Chris, why is it raining? You're the weatherman, damn it! It's supposed to be sunny in Miami. Why is it raining?"

Then he'd whack the kid or yank his hair so hard that a handful came out or pick up something and fire it at Chris. Everyone got hit at Columbus. It was almost an entertainment form for both teachers and students. The ones being hurt usually provided a good laugh for everyone else, so the pain produced a dose of fun.

At Christmas, we were "encouraged" to bring teachers bottles of booze as presents. It was understood that the better the quality of booze, the greater the grade increase. Given our savvy for exploiting every available opportunity, many of us submitted one bottle for extra credit and kept another for our own holiday cheer. Obviously, our parents would support any extra credit by willfully providing us with as much liquor as we needed. Let me boil it down for you: On the last day before the Christmas holidays, teachers' desks were covered with spirits, and students were basically drunk during school hours. Hallelujah!!

Even though I had much more fun in high school, I didn't do any better in the classroom. I earned mostly Cs and Ds with a few Bs and a couple Fs. I managed an A in history with the teacher who threw things at us. I liked that teacher in spite of his approach to discipline. As a result, I did well in his class. If I liked the subject, or the teacher, or both, then I usually did well. I went on to earn an A in Florida history, and another one in world history in subsequent years.

Math was just the opposite; it was very, very difficult for me. There were points when I tried, but I just didn't understand math. Maybe I didn't think about it to the extent I should have. Either way, they just kept jamming it down my throat. I went to summer school for math. I had more tutors. Still I wondered: Why wouldn't they encourage me to focus on my strengths rather than put all the attention on my deficiencies? It made no sense.

Then again, it was a different time, to say the least. The summer between my freshman and sophomore years our head football coach, Bob Lewis, took a bunch of boys on a camping and hiking trip in the

Canadian Rockies. There were ten or twelve of us in one of those small school vans. Lewis drove us from Miami through the western United States, through North Dakota and up into Canada in that thing. We went to Yellowstone, Mt. Rushmore, and Glacier National Park. We were gone for a month.

In Atikokan, a small town in Canada, we were outfitted with canoes and camping gear before embarking on a 150-mile adventure. We hiked and canoed every day, moving twenty miles or so before stopping to set up camp. We were kids so of course we were screwing around. One morning, Lewis told us he had enough, and we could find our own way home. He just jumped in a canoe and paddled away.

Think about that. Here we were, a bunch of kids in the middle of nowhere, and the guy just leaves. Everyone was freaking out, but I didn't care. Not only did I have the map, but I had spent years in summer camp in North Carolina and central Florida learning survival skills. I also earned a Master's Certificate in canoeing. We packed up all our stuff and started paddling down the river. About five miles from the camp, we found the guy. If that happened today, he would still be in jail. But that's how it was back then. You learned to fend for yourself and, for the most part, it was a great way to grow up.

We would come to know Coach Lewis had some issues. In my junior year, we had a great football team—arguably one of the best in Columbus's history. I earned the starting position at middle line-backer, the same position my brother played during his high school career. Mike Shula was our quarterback and Alonzo Highsmith, who became an All-America running back at the University of Miami, and the third pick of the 1987 NFL draft, played defensive end. He was considered the best high school athlete in the country. Midway through the season, our defensive coordinator called a team meeting to tell us Coach Lewis had resigned. Later that evening, I learned the truth behind his sudden departure. I was getting ready to go out for the night when a friend of mine, whose brother worked at the *Miami Herald*, came to our house and broke the news that would be all over the front page of the newspaper the next morning. Our coach had been arrested for "lewd and lascivious behavior" in the company of another man the previous night on Watson Island, near Miami Beach.

Here we were, an all-boys Catholic school with a great football team, and our head coach literally got caught with his pants down. It was huge news all over South Florida, and it was embarrassing for everyone. The ridicule, jokes, and razzing followed us all over town and all through the football season.

The only place we could answer all the comments was on the football field. I don't know if it was to prove a point, or whether we were just scared to lose, but we didn't lose a game until we made it to the state championship.

Even great success on the football field couldn't dull the stress around school—particularly when it came to grades. Eventually, I just didn't care. The night before a test can be stressful for most kids. Not me. I went to bed the night before a test without ever cracking a book. I slept like a baby. I remained a happy-go-lucky kid, stress or no stress.

It wasn't like I didn't have great examples at home. My parents never gave us money unless we earned it. You want to go to the movies? Clean the pool, weed the garden, or trim the bushes; nothing came easily or free. Besides, I had a lifestyle to maintain with girl-friends. I could always use extra cash. That's the motivation that drove a lot of what my friends and I did, including some stealing, some of which could have gotten us into serious trouble. We were always doing pranks, nothing serious initially.

Some of the guys I was hanging out with, not necessarily my close friends, had an advanced sense of mischief. For instance, I was in charge of the bottle room at a local grocery store. When someone turned in a six-gallon water bottle, they received a five- or six-dol-lar refund. I would turn in bottles that had already been turned in to collect another five or six dollars for myself. Since I knew where the bottles were kept, I'd go to another store in the chain, walk right into the back room, pick up three or four bottles and take them to the counter, and "return" them. That would be twenty or twenty-four dollars right there, enough for a date in those days, without having to clean the pool or trim the bushes.

I also was in charge of taking out the garbage at the grocery store, which presented another opportunity for mischief and personal gain.

I'd throw cases of beer and packages of steaks into the garbage. Later after work, I'd go behind the building and dig out my loot.

It wasn't a matter of trying to avoid work. I always had a job. I worked from the time I was fifteen years old. I worked for a couple years in the grocery store. I worked for a pizza parlor as a busboy—cleaning tables and washing dishes. I was a hamburger cook at Fuddrucker's, a camp counselor, and a fisherman. I didn't work during the football season, but I usually had a job the rest of the school year. I might not have been the model student, but I put a lot of effort into making sure the last four years of my education were a lot more fun than the first eight.

Columbus High School is no longer the country club that it was in the early 1980s. The Marist Brothers have done a tremendous job making it a wonderful learning establishment, with incredible amounts of resources for the students to thrive. I am truly proud to say that I am a Columbus Explorer. Wherever I go, I always run into fellow Columbus alums. When you come from a brotherhood like that, you know it was a special place.

Chapter 8

Life After Football

DAD: The first contact I had with U.S. Tobacco (UST) was at a cocktail party in Miami. They brought their biggest customers to Doral, a well-known and respected golf community in South Florida. The event was called "What Are You Doing New Year's Eve?" which was the theme of the party they threw every year. That year they took everyone to the Orange Bowl to watch a college bowl game.

The company called the Dolphins and requested four players to attend the cocktail party and spend a couple hours mingling and signing autographs. They paid us $1,500 each, which was amazing. Back then in 1973, I was probably making $75,000 a year playing football. This is after being All-Pro seven or eight times and playing in two Super Bowls.

When the two hours were over, the rest of the guys went home. I stayed. I really hit it off with the CEO, and I had a really good time at the event. I was talking to the executives, and they invited me to dinner. In the course of the conversation, they said, "What are you doing in February? We have our National Association of Tobacco and Candy Distributors Convention at the Fontainebleau in Miami Beach."

I said, "I'm available and I'd be happy to do it."

"How about if we signed you to a contract, and you can do some other things for us too?"

I brought pictures that I autographed for a long line of people. After the Fontainebleau event they said, "Look, we'd like to sign you to a three-year contract to come to our events." They offered me $25,000 per year, which was amazing. Then they went out and signed Walt Garrison of the Dallas Cowboys, Earl Campbell from the Houston Oilers, Bobby Murcer from the New York Yankees, and Shep Messing, who was a soccer goalie. We had a ball. From there the relationship mushroomed.

You have to remember that endorsements didn't amount to much in the early 1970s. Being paid $1,000 to speak at a banquet in Chicago was a lot of money. We didn't have anybody marketing us the way athletes do today. It was found money, and it was good money. The opportunity developed into a phenomenal relationship. My secretary, Barbara Shaver, who was with me for nearly thirty years until she passed away in 2009, always said, "You always seem to take advantage of the situation at precisely the right time."

I was a practicing attorney in Miami, and I was doing some work for the Florida Tobacco and Candy Association. That meant I was pretty much intertwined with the tobacco business. It was consistent with my background because the first job I ever had was as an eleven-year-old on a tobacco farm. I worked tobacco for two years. The bus picked me up at 5:30 in the morning and dropped me back home at 3 o'clock in the afternoon. It was the dirtiest, filthiest job you can imagine. I worked in Southwick, Massachusetts. There are still tobacco farms there. They grow the outer leaf for cigars. Later, when I was playing with the Patriots, I worked for a tobacco-candy distributor called Garber Bros. Paul Garber became a good friend and he hired me. I got to know the business a little bit.

When I started practicing law and doing work for the Candy and Tobacco Association, UST brought me to a couple meetings, and they were impressed with what they saw. They hired me on an annual basis. I was making more money with them than I was playing football. It was a hell of a bonus to my income. Then, when I retired, they continued me on a contract that increased every year.

In 1978 the company, which was headquartered in Greenwich, Connecticut, asked me to become Corporate Secretary. Terry and I looked at schools in Connecticut. I did my homework. I brought everything home, and we analyzed the entire decision as a family. At the time, Gina was going into her senior year in high school, Nicky was a junior and a good football player, and Marc was heading into eighth grade. I got everyone together in the dining room.

It was a hell of a decision. The only one who voted for the move was Marc. I found out later that he had ulterior motives, which wasn't surprising. Terry was willing to go, but it wasn't the right time to move. I turned down the job. It was unusual and certainly not something people would do today. But I respected the fact that the kids had all their friendships in Miami, and we didn't have to move.

Instead of turning their backs on me, UST offered me a position on their board. That's when I started corporate life. Then a couple years later, they offered me the position of Sr. Vice President, which was a bigger job with a lot more money. At the time, I had a very good law practice. I was representing National Council on Compensation Insurance, which represented all the workman's compensation companies in the state of Florida. The Tobacco and Candy Association was a client, and I had ten or twelve baseball players I represented—among them were Bucky Dent, Mickey Rivers, Andre Dawson, Warren Cromartie, Ron Davis, and Dave Righetti, and a few football players like Nat Moore, who played for the Dolphins. I had a good practice so I didn't need to go corporate.

The practice was building, and I was doing a good job for my clients. When I first started I had a partner, Barry Garber, who became a federal judge in Miami. His practice was so different from my practice that we finally split the firm. He did a lot of criminal law. I was more on the civil side doing commercial law. It was really just Barbara, who was my right hand, and me. A couple of young guys came to work for me as interns along the way. One of them was Rick Horrow, who is now one of the premier consultants on stadium construction in the country. The other guy who interned with me was Drew Rosenhaus, who has become one of the most successful agents in the NFL.

The agent part of the business started to change as the players became more demanding. Some of them no longer thought about the fact I had a life of my own. As a result, it became something that was no longer desirable on my part. My favorite saying to my sports clients was, "You play the game. I'll take care of the money." And I did.

When Andre Dawson was a young player with the Montreal Expos I had a meeting on Atlantic Avenue in Delray Beach with John McHale, who was general manager of the team. Andre wasn't even eligible for arbitration. I got him his first million-dollar contract. That's when a million dollars was a lot of money.

Back then guys were better to deal with. Nowadays contracts are pretty much spelled out. There isn't as much room to finesse and negotiate. I'm not so sure guys can't negotiate their own deals at this point, particularly in the NBA and NFL. There's no magic to the process these days as terms are spelled out in collective bargaining agreements.

The point is, the offer UST made had to be significant for me to move, which it was. So, I took the job in 1983, and moved to Greenwich. By then, Nicky was at Duke and Gina was at the University of Florida. Marc was heading into his senior year at Columbus. He stayed behind with Terry, but I flew home most weekends.

When I went to work for UST it was the right decision in the long run—more right than I could have imagined at the time for reasons no one could have foreseen.

Chapter 9

Older and Bolder

By the time I was a senior in high school, my dad had climbed even higher up the corporate ladder at UST. As a result, I had more freedom. My father spent three weeks out of the month in Connecticut, and my mom went up once or twice a month to stay with him. That left me home alone, in Miami in the 1980s, with all the necessary resources—cars, connections, and money to survive on.

Eventually, I started hanging out with some guys who were a little more hard-core than my childhood friends. My friends were fun, but they were also loving, good people. The guys I was spending time with during my senior year pushed the limits on most everything. The pranks became more daring, the risks more dangerous.

Some of the characters I was running around with went to school with me; others I met through them. Many of them had older brothers. As a result, they were relatively advanced when it came to pushing the edges of the law. In terms of drugs and violence, there was so much going on at that time in Miami. Our actions mirrored the times. I was sixteen years old the summer before my senior year, and I went to parties every weekend. For example, some of the guys I was with would go into the other rooms of the house where the party was taking place looking for the girls' purses. Even though it was wrong, there was a perverse psychological lure to it all because of the risk involved.

It was the thrill of the hunt combined with the fact that everyone was acquiring expensive lifestyles or habits in some cases. Whether it was buying nice clothes or acquiring things to enhance our recreational experiences, there wasn't a great deal of guilt or conscience involved. All that Catholic guilt we had been fed lost its effectiveness somewhere along the way. We were no longer concerned with "right and wrong." All we cared about was not getting caught.

There were many nights when I lay awake in my room worried about the wrong car showing up at my house. I didn't know if that car would have police lights on top of it or a bunch of bad guys showing up with weapons. There was at least one occasion when I feared the police less than a group of guys from the other side of town. There was once a huge guy from another high school in Miami who was rumored to have wanted to kill me.

Let's just say, I had the potential of getting into serious criminal trouble. A bunch of us were inches from getting caught for stealing one time. Someone stole a credit card at a party. The next day we went to a surf shop to buy surfboards. What no one knew is that some surfboards don't come with the fins. You have to buy the fins separately and screw them into the bottom of the board. One of the guys sent a couple girls back into the store to buy the fins. By that time, the shop manager had figured out the credit cards were bogus. When the girls came out they were scared to death because the manager started asking them all kinds of questions. I was on the other side of the mall at the time. The girls weren't very smart. They probably didn't know the surfboards were effectively stolen three days earlier when we had taken the credit cards. Everyone disappeared as soon as the girls came out of the store.

I was standing by myself when the two guys from the store started walking toward me. I just turned around and started walking down the street. Finally, I stopped and yelled, "What?" I was ready to fight both of them. "Why are you guys following me?"

"We don't want any trouble," one of them said. "Just give us the surfboards back."

"I don't know what you're talking about, man. I'm not giving anything back. But if you keep following me, you're going to get a fat lip."

They ended up leaving and I just kept walking until I saw my friend's car. We could have ended up in serious trouble. They could have called the police and fairly easily identified at least one of us. All they needed was one name.

The kinds of things I was doing were 180 degrees from the expectations of our household. My mother was effectively a cop and the rules were mercilessly enforced. I used a lot of eye drops, chewed a lot of gum, and regularly doused cologne to cover up the pot smell, or the alcohol. My mother always told my father, "Your son is on drugs." I don't think my dad wanted to acknowledge the idea that his son was experimenting. That's all it really was in terms of drugs, though. I smoked pot, but that was like stealing a sip from your mother's wine glass compared to what was going on in Miami in the 1980s. It wasn't uncommon to see bales of pot floating in Biscayne Bay or even a drug plane landing on a highway.

Through it all, I never got in real trouble. I was pulled over by the police three different times while someone in the car was smoking pot. I was let go every time. I'm sure my name had something do to with it, but so did the times. I do remember one time my name coming up as an officer looked over my license.

"Oh, one of Nick's sons. What are you doing?"

"Smoking a joint, sir."

"Don't let me catch you smoking again."

That was it.

My mother knew what was going on. Like every mother, she had that special radar to detect anything even slightly out of order. One time she told me, "I'm going out of town. Do not use my car." She had a brand-new BMW, which was parked in the garage with the keys available. Needless to say, I used her car. Everything was fine except I lost my rolling papers somewhere in the car. I searched every inch of that vehicle trying to find them before my mother returned home. Within minutes of getting into her car, she found them. Not only was I busted for taking the car, but she also realized what I had been doing.

In the end, it was kind of funny, at least to me, because she found the rolling papers.

"Well, they *are* made by U.S. Tobacco," I noted, "so at least I'm supporting the company brand."

To put my habits in perspective, my idol at the time was Bob Marley. He died of cancer in Miami at Cedar's of Lebanon Hospital. Bob's mother was Cedella Booker, and I knew one of her children from another father. I grew up with the Bookers, Richard and Anthony, as well as Bob's son Rohan Marley, who played football at Palmetto High and later at the University of Miami. One day Anthony ended up being shot to death. He went to the Cutler Ridge Mall (now Southland Mall) wearing a bulletproof vest and carrying a shotgun. Something happened to him, either some bad drugs or mental illness, because he was the kindest guy you could ever meet. After recklessly wielding a weapon in the open mall, he was shot to death by an off-duty police officer.

I knew Julian Marley too. In college, after my injury, I managed a reggae band with Johnny Guardiola ("Johnny Dread"), a Cuban friend from high school. I even produced an album that did very well. I had my own record label, Marcus Records, and the band was called Copacetic.

I never met Bob, but I met Rita Marley, Bob's wife, and a lot of the Marley kids. I played basketball with all the Wailers. A friend, Will Holstrum, lived across the street from Bob and Rita. I used to keep my motorcycle at Will's house because my parents forbade me to have one. Not only did my parents never know that I had a Kawasaki 175, but it was probably stolen. I paid some guy a hundred dollars for the bike.

That's how I met the Marleys. They were always outside playing basketball so Will and I would go across the street and play with them. Bob died in 1981 and I didn't start hanging around his mom's house until 1983 or so. That was part of my connection to reggae. I remember loving Rita's song "One Draw," and it all came together for me. I was rebellious, they were singing about smoking weed, and it was all about having a good time, which was pretty much exactly what I was about at the time. Besides, I really liked the music.

It was a great experience to spend time with the original reggae family. I smoked pot with Cedella as we listened to her son playing on a tape. She even rolled the joint with her own hands. It was beautiful. Smoking pot with Bob Marley's mom? Come on, how can you do better than that?

My grandparents were around and they would check on me from time to time, but I was on my own a lot as a high school senior. I got myself up for school every morning, and I never missed a day. I actually enjoyed school at Columbus even though I was a poor student. I would be late here and there, and I played the angles to be sure, but I was responsible when it came to showing up for class. Of course, I had a few tricks up my sleeve for this as well. For example, I knew that the first note I brought to school at the beginning of the year was one they had on file to compare future signatures against. Most kids didn't realize that so they were caught whenever they tried to sneak through a fake note.

I was so adept at the process that early in my senior year I had my friend Rick Arango—who had handwriting like a girl—write a note on my behalf. It read simply, "To whom it may concern. Please excuse my son Marc from being late. He had a dentist appointment. Terry Buoniconti." So I handed in my note early in the year, and I was good to go. One time I had a real dentist appointment. What's funny is that I couldn't use the note my mother wrote. Her handwriting didn't match Rick's. I had to have Rick create a forgery of a real note!

Another one of my friends, Jose Puig, had an aunt who was maybe five years older than us. She had a Cuban accent, but she would call into the school for us if we were late, or skipping a few classes. The school never said a word. She would call in and say, "This is Mrs. Buoniconti. Please excuse my son Marc, he is going to the dentist today." She was twenty-one years old with a heavy accent, and I was perfectly comfortable passing her off as my mother. I was careful, though, when I used these options.

In my mind, angles existed for a reason—to be played.

Funny thing, Rick, Jose, and I formed the triumvirate that pulled off possibly the most daring and legendary prank of our times. Like many questionable acts this one, too, began with a dare. Over a game of bocce ball, Jose's brother-in-law, Bob Pardo, shared with us past lore of his involvement in an alleged streaking incident ten years before at the all-girls Our Lady of Lourdes Academy, the sister school to Columbus. Bob claimed that he and some of his friends had pulled off the reprehensible act of exposing themselves to Catholic schoolgirls and nuns. This was all we needed to hear. Sadly, even after all those years of Catholic education, there wasn't a moment of hesitation in me. I was only interested in the lure of excitement and the promise of legendary status.

The execution involved a preliminary stakeout of the school and a map detailing our route, complete with a getaway car driven by another schoolmate named Alex Gutierrez. It went down on a Friday when we had a half-day of classes. We knew the girls at Lourdes had a full day of classes. We strategically positioned ourselves across the street from the main entrance wearing only shorts and sneakers, ski masks in hand.

"Are we doing this?" The question was asked as if a glimmer of consciousness might prevail.

"Hell yeah, we're doing it!" I exclaimed.

And, to ward off any further doubt, off went my shorts, on went the mask, and away we went—with nothing to lose and everything to lose. It was two minutes of fury—girls screaming and nuns yelling—classic!

But loose lips sink ships. Even though we had done our best to keep the act covert, and we escaped unscathed, we paid the price the following Monday. The afternoon announcements began just like any other day. For a second I thought we might get away with it. Just then, moments before dismissal, the voice of Lou Savino, our dean of discipline, blasted over the loudspeakers, "The following people report to my office: Rick Arango, Marc Buoniconti, and Jose Puig." Mr. Savino was well known for general intimidation and liberal use of corporal punishment. The three of us arrived just outside his office.

"Get in here! What made you feel the need to expose yourselves to women who had dedicated their entire lives to God?"

To our great astonishment, the punishment was no more than one Saturday detention. We chalked that up to an act of Catholic forgiveness.

The streaking, like so many of my exploits, only added fuel to the fire, in particular between my mom and me. The constant butting of heads and battle of wills culminated in my packing a bag and leaving home to escape her. The grinding rigidity of her rules and my free spirit brought my home life to a halt. I went to stay at my friend Jamie Anderson's house for four or five days. He lived in the neighborhood, and his mom was extremely lenient. I'm sure my mom knew where I was. She knew I was going to school every day, that's for sure.

I couldn't take it anymore. It took an intercession by my principal, Brother Edmund Sheehan, to bring us to the bargaining table. My parents, Brother Sheehan, and I sat in our living room as each of them ran off their list of disappointments. Believe me, I wanted to come home every night. I missed my mother. I realized that all she really wanted was the best for me. A truce was reached. I agreed to tone it down. She would do her best to loosen the vise. I agreed to come home with one thing in mind: make it to graduation.

Chapter 10

Our Wild Child

DAD: Of course I was worried about Marc. His grades were terrible. He was wild. It's not that we treated him any differently than our other kids. We disciplined him the same way we did Nicky and Gina.

Terry was a taskmaster. She was really involved in the kids' lives. Her parents were alive then, and they were very involved too. I was involved in their lives, coaching softball and baseball. Marc just had a wild hair that couldn't be managed. I can remember the days when we knew he needed a 2.0 average to graduate from high school. We didn't know whether he was going to graduate. He'd say, "Dad, don't worry about it. I've got it made." He knew because he had done the calculations and figured it all out. He knew that if he earned a C in religion that would be enough to graduate.

I don't think there was any academic curriculum that would have made him study at that time. If you asked him to put together his own curriculum, I'm not sure it would have been possible for him to find something other than sports, fishing, diving, and a lot of other things, that interested him enough to make him study.

Marc was always very confident, cocky in some ways. He knew exactly what he was doing. He would tell us not to worry about him, that he was doing fine. He had my confidence, but he had a sense of arrogance too.

He felt like he was above the system. Once you get to that point, where you think you are above the system, that's when you run into difficulty. People who are in the system working hard to accomplish things don't understand someone who puts himself above the law, the rules, and regulations. That's what holds society together.

It was Marc who came to us with the idea of attending The Citadel. He said, "Dad I need the discipline. That's probably the only place where I won't flunk out. I need to go to military school." It shocked the hell out of me. Kids can grow up in the same house, but they don't all have the same genes. Look at the people who send their kids off to private schools. They expect that child to come home well-educated, disciplined, courteous, kind, and considerate. The first thing they do once they come home from school is crack up the car because they were out drinking. That's what happens when you bring up children. I think it's the nature of the beast. It's a crapshoot.

I was pretty much intent on him going to prep school; that's what he should have done. When The Citadel came around I couldn't believe Marc wanted to do it. Unlike Nicky, who was choosing between Dartmouth and Duke, Marc didn't have any schools knocking his door down. Back then it wasn't like it is today. I don't think the coaches were doing a lot of placement like they do now. Marc was one of the best players in the state, but he wasn't academically qualified for most schools.

* * *

MOM: I thought Marc would either be in jail or dead by the time he was twenty.

Nick never knew how bad Marc was because Nick was away in Connecticut. I would tell him, "Marc is using pot. He's not doing well in school. We have a problem here."

Nick just didn't want to believe me. He didn't want to come home after being away for weeks at a time and have to yell at Marc. He didn't want to recognize that we really did have a problem. I'm Catholic and I still have calluses on my knees from all the praying for Marc. Him alone!

Marc always had pretty girlfriends and people would tell me what a nice young man he was, but Marc was a hellion. When I say I had calluses on my knees, I'm not kidding. I got to the point with Marc that I went to church every single day. When Nicky and Gina were off at college and it was just Marc and me at home, oh boy. He ran away at least once, and I threw him out several other times.

I was involved at Columbus too. They had the athletic club and I was involved in raising money. I was there a lot. I knew his grades weren't very good. The Brothers were a little better about keeping the parents informed about what was happening in school. Of course, Marc was at school every Saturday painting or cleaning up because of detentions. When it came time for college, he wanted to play football. His last head coach said he couldn't recommend Marc because he was a discipline problem. What did I think would happen? Jail. But Marc never worried. He was confident he'd end up somewhere.

To put his high school years in perspective, I didn't find out he would graduate until the night before the ceremony on Baccalaureate night. I went to Brother Angelo, who taught Marc English. I looked at him and said, "Well, Brother?"

He looked back and said, "Barely."

That's how I found out Marc was actually going to graduate from high school. Until that moment, I didn't know whether or not he was going to get a blank diploma when they called his name at graduation. He didn't know either.

I was so happy The Citadel came along because no one else would take him. Marc was an incredible ballplayer. He just had a feel for the game. When The Citadel came along I thought, "Thank you, God. A military school!"

When we brought him there, and I started to really understand the process, I wasn't sure whether Marc would make it through.

Chapter 11

Going Commando

My focus was on football, and I figured football would take care of me. In retrospect, my thought process was more than a little misguided. What do you expect? I saw myself being written about in the *Miami Herald* and other newspapers. As a senior I was named All-County, then All-State. I was chosen one of the twelve best football players in Miami-Dade County. To me, it seemed reasonable to expect football would bail me out. I knew my grades were awful, but I also knew I could play at a high level.

During the season, my coach tolerated me. But as time went on, he saw what a screw-up I was. He knew I was all about having a good time, which was the polar opposite of him. He was a conservative Catholic, salt of the earth kind of guy. He saw right through me. I would be playing Frisbee, getting a suntan in the parking lot, shirtless with sunglasses—remember this is a Catholic school that required shirt and tie—when I should have been in class. He knew. He might not have known everything I was doing, but he knew enough.

We went to the state championship game for the second time in school history my junior year, both times with a Buoniconti as the team's starting middle linebacker. Still, my coach didn't like what I did off the field, and he certainly didn't like what I did in his classroom. He felt differently about me when I was on the field.

An article in the *Miami Herald* compared my style to the way my dad played with the Dolphins. Here's what my coach had to say about me then in that article, which was a lot nicer than what he said to me after my senior season: "It's uncanny how similar they are, especially their intensity. Neither one is theoretically big enough to be great at the levels they play at, but what makes them better is their relentlessness. It's their heart that separates them from the other players around them." Unbeknownst to me at that time, these words would prove to be prophetic.

After my junior season, I received letters from everywhere, including: Oklahoma, Duke, Georgia, Penn State, Louisville, Mississippi State, East Carolina, and South Carolina. These were big schools with great football programs. We went 8-2 my senior year. I received even more letters from just about every major football program. But I never got beyond the letters. From what I later came to understand, when schools contacted my coach, he told all of them to stay away from me. He told them I had an attitude problem, among other things. Maybe he was trying to save face for himself. He didn't want to recommend me, and then have me screw up everything and make him look bad. I suppose he was half-right. I had an attitude problem, but not on the field.

The University of Miami coaches saw me play, but I wasn't very big. I was a five-foot-eleven, 190-pound middle linebacker in high school. I might have been a great player at that level, but I'm sure some schools, even without the other issues, wondered about my ability to play at the next level. You would think the fact that my brother was starting middle linebacker at Duke University, and my dad having done what he did, would have made schools give me a second look. And maybe they did. I don't know. Despite all the letters, The Citadel was the only school to me make me an offer.

Part of it was my fault because I only filled out a few applications. I think I sent one to Eastern Carolina, the University of Kansas, and maybe Boston College. The truth is that I might not have sent any because I probably didn't want to take the time to go through the process. That just shows you where I was at the time. I figured they would want me so they would come and find me. That's how I thought it worked. I knew something was fishy, though, when Syracuse University recruiters came to Columbus one day after the season. I mentioned to my coach that I heard they would be in the building that day. His response: "They won't be interested in you."

When our football season ended, the coaches called all the senior players into a meeting about recruiting. Our head coach walked us through the process, how it worked. Then, one by one he went through the team, and talked about who would get a scholarship, the level of the school it might come from, and what each player should expect. He didn't say a word about me or my friend Rick Arango, who was an excellent player. Rick and I got into a lot of trouble together. We had a great time in high school, all of which our coach knew.

Still, our high school team was loaded with talent, and we were two of the best players. Rick ended up playing at the University of Miami. Dwayne Ganzy went to Syracuse, Bill Mendoza to Marshall, Scott DiMare to Florida State, and Carlos Avalos went to The Citadel. So every college recruiter had seen me play. I was the team captain. I led the team in tackles and came close to leading in interceptions. I was voted the team's Most Valuable Player. They knew what I could do on the football field but it didn't matter.

When the meeting ended, our coach looked at Rick and me.

"You two stay right here."

He shut the door and the first thing out of his mouth was, "I'm going to put the fucking cards on the table right now! You two have made a mockery of your senior year!"

He pointed to Rick and said, "I don't know what you're doing hanging out with Buoniconti. He's a loser. You guys had all the potential in the world."

He was right about the last part. He ended the speech by telling me, "I don't even know why a school like The Citadel would want you, Buoniconti. It's your final chance but I know you, and you're going to fuck that up too. You're going to be back here with your tail between your legs in two months."

That's the kind of guy he was. To some extent I don't blame him, though we were still kids. But I will say that ironically enough that talk is one of the reasons I refused to buckle at The Citadel. I wanted to prove him and everyone else wrong.

When Rick and I walked out of the meeting room, we looked at one other and said, "Oh, shit." Rick was a good student until he started hanging around with me. He had a 3.0 every year until his senior year, when he barely finished with a 2.0. Nonetheless, I'm pretty sure that after the deliberations we proceeded to get high.

I had never even heard of The Citadel the day the school's football recruiter came to Columbus. I went into the coach's office and there was one of my game tapes up on the reel. The recruiter told me I was the kind of player The Citadel wanted. He was young and a good guy, with a bit of a surfer-beach look. We connected right away. He told me where the school was located and talked about what a great city Charleston, South Carolina, was and how much I would like going to school there. He didn't say much about the school's culture. I did a little research and found out it was a military college, but I had no idea what was in store for me.

My mother saw the uniforms the cadets wore and instantly thought the idea of me going to The Citadel was wonderful. At the time, I was dating a girl whose father was retired Navy, so The Citadel was an easy choice, especially when the only other choice I had was prep school.

I took my only college visit to The Citadel. In retrospect, during that visit they covered up a lot in terms of what life was like for freshmen. I was taken care of by upperclassmen, football players. They were my chaperones for the weekend. I spent very little time on campus. They took me to The Citadel Beach House and to downtown Charleston to hang out with some alumni. The school had just built a new football facility, and we spent a lot of time there as well. They showed me the battalions. They took me into the regimental commander's room—the highest ranked cadet on campus who is assigned the nicest and largest room—so I could see how nice the rooms were, which was totally misleading. His room was not only three times larger than the other rooms, but he had a television and a telephone. It seemed great at the time. Of course, I didn't know freshmen weren't allowed to have a telephone, and no one was allowed to have a television until their senior year.

I also didn't see the rest of life at The Citadel. I didn't see freshmen being screamed at or otherwise abused by upperclassmen. I didn't see anybody marching, no hazing, nothing that might have soured me on the school. They focused on the beautiful football facility, the wonderful quarters of the regimental commander, and Charleston, which is a great city. Not to mention the fact that I managed to hook up with two different girls the nights I stayed in Charleston. I thought to myself, "How bad can it be?"

One of the players said, "There's a little bit of discipline, a little bit of marching, but nothing to worry about. It's not that bad. You'll love it at The Citadel." Besides, The Citadel coach called me every week or so leading up to signing day. So I signed.

I thought about going to prep school to get my grades up because I was young. My birthday is in late September, so I was a year younger than just about everyone else in my class growing up. I was only sixteen when I started my senior year of high school and seventeen a month into my freshman year of college. I was still a growing kid.

At the same time, I really felt like a burden on my parents and my family. I was rebellious and very independent. I'm not proud of a lot of what I did in high school, but that's who I was at the time. The fact I had a scholarship sealed the deal. I would no longer be a bother to my parents. I wouldn't need their money, either. That's how I found my way to The Citadel. We had a very close family, but I had an independent streak. The scholarship provided me a way to break free, and to prove to everyone and myself that despite my maladjusted behavior and misguided decision-making, in the end, I earned a football scholarship on my own.

Chapter 12

F-Troop

A couple days before I left for The Citadel I heard that one of the first things they do to freshmen is shave their heads. I thought it would be a good idea to get ahead of the game, or at least appear to be in control of the situation. So Dodie helped me shave my head.

When I first arrived on campus, I immediately went over to the locker room at the football facility for a welcome reception with all the other freshmen scholarship players. Everything seemed fine. The head coach, Tom Moore, introduced us to the coaching staff, and we all mingled, sharing some time to get acquainted. Our defensive coordinator, Billy Smith, who went on to coach in the NFL, gave the defensive players a spirited pep talk. We then broke into our linebackers meeting with our position coach, Will Holthauser. The first thing he did was to put a big pinch of Copenhagen chewing tobacco in his mouth. I felt comfortable right away.

After all the pleasantries were over, we were all lined up again. Then we were sent off to our respective battalions and dormitories. The dorm facility was something you had to see to believe. It looked like a prison. In fact, a prison looked more welcoming. There was a large parade ground in the center of campus, surrounded by similar looking white castle design structures, each with parapet moldings.

All the buildings were lined up in meticulous order as if standing at attention. On the west side of the parade ground stood four-square buildings and one big rectangular building, my new home. That's where my battalion resided.

Second Battalion was the worst place to be, not only because it was the largest of the four battalions, but it also housed the toughest companies, and was where all the executive officers lived. A "company" is a military term for a subdivision of a regiment or battalion. Each company is made up of approximately one hundred cadets of equal numbers of freshmen, sophomores, juniors, and seniors.

Second Battalion housed four companies; mine was called F-Troop. In addition to the regimental commander and his staff, every company was structured with a cadet system that follows the military chain of command. That's military jargon for, if they outrank you, you're screwed! "Upperclassmen" are basically those cadets who survived their freshman year. Sophomores have extremely limited privileges, juniors a bit more, and seniors can actually enjoy moments of relaxation not dissimilar to inmates in a federal prison. Freshmen have absolutely no privileges and are considered lower than the lowest form of scum. It is the duty of the upperclassmen to "shape" and "mold" the freshmen into model cadets who personify the virtues and honor of the institution. All that meant was that the relationship between the upperclassmen and freshmen was reducible to the simple formula: "Now that we're not freshmen, let's torture the hell out of them." Not all, but most upperclassmen lived to mess with freshmen. The incoming sophomores were the worst. They had just finished the previous year as freshmen. They had been licking their chops all summer long waiting for payback. We were like raw meat about to be thrown to the lions. Of course, I saw none of that on my recruiting trip. What came next I probably wouldn't have believed anyway.

When I arrived at Second Battalion, I was still in jeans and as far as I knew I was just going to be settling in. I had all my things in a bag. Again, my point of reference was the recruiting weekend. I had no idea what was about to happen. We walked into the gate and there were officers around us. No big deal. I don't know if they thought I was an upperclassman because my head was already shaved, but initially no one said much to me. Then, all of a sudden, two or three guys walked up to us and realized that we were freshmen. It was like somebody flipped a switch. These guys went completely berserk. They were right up to the edge of being completely out of control.

"Get your face up against that wall!" one of them yelled.

"The party is over!"

"Your momma isn't here to save you!"

"We're going to break you!"

"By the end of the day you'll wish you had never been born!"

"Now get on your face and start doing push-ups until I tell you to stop!"

My immediate and only thought: "What did I get myself into?"

"Get on your feet right now!"

"Stand at attention!"

We were flustered and fumbling around. They just kept screaming. "Eyes front! Don't look at me!" I was kind of laughing inside because I had no idea what was going on. But it didn't stop. For the next thirty minutes these guys just kept screaming. They put us in formation as they tried to teach us how to salute properly.

The minute a new guy came into the room, it started all over again. We stood in line and it was wild, a complete shock. Every one of those guys would get right in your face and yell "the party's over, knob!" invoking the tradition of referring to our shaved heads as the door knobs they resembled. And the yelling would resume. "Your life is over! Don't think you can go cry to your momma! Your ass is ours now! One hour with me and you'll all quit!" All the while they're spitting in our faces. Now I'm really thinking: "Oh my God . . ."

And it didn't stop for eight months, the same intensity all day, every day. Later on, I realized those initial moments were tame compared to what would follow.

Another guy from South Florida lasted just two weeks. He left before school even started. I wasn't entirely alone. One of my Columbus teammates, Carlos Avalos, was there. But they split us up right away, putting us in separate companies and battalions.

The upperclassmen ran us into our rooms to drop off our things. They made us change into shorts and a T-shirt. Then they ran us all into another area. They put what they called an "idiot bag" around our necks. It was a plastic bag with The Citadel Guide, which contained all the military and institutional crap we had to memorize and recite at a moment's notice. Basically, everything you needed to know was in that book. You had to learn The Citadel prayer, the cadet song, all the rules, the rifle maneuvers, everything. Now, this is still two weeks before the arrival of the rest of the students. This two-week period is strictly for the freshmen football players to give us time to adjust and start learning the basics.

Initially, I was shocked and flustered because guys were screaming at me and no one knew what to do. That first day was a blur. They lined up the freshmen football players together in shorts, T-shirts, idiot bags, black shoes, and black socks. We looked like morons. We were in formation, and guys were trying to teach us how to march, how to stand at attention and brace. Bracing is standing at attention with your arms pressed tightly against your sides, shoulders rolled back, and chin tucked into your chest, locked in hard. You have to squeeze your fists and hold your arms locked against your body as tightly as you can.

While you're doing that, the upperclassmen come by and pull on your arms. If they can pull your arms away from your sides, then it's down on the ground for push-ups. That was bracing. We did it all day. Eventually we went to get our uniforms, and there was a whole process related to uniforms as well. They taught us where the name tag went, how to shine our shoes, how to shine the brass. All of this happened on the first day. And you had to get it all down that day because there was no more teaching after that. They just expected you to know everything.

Finally, at 11 p.m., we got to our rooms, which involved another new process. They told us how to keep our clothes. Everything had to be hung up in a very specific way. Clothes not meant for hangers had to be folded correctly, and put into the drawer. There was a specific way to make the bed. Everything was by the book, a book with no exceptions.

It was after midnight by the time we were able to go to sleep. It was the first opportunity I had to introduce myself to my roommate,

George Thomas. We didn't say much, mostly because we didn't have the energy. It was more like, "Do you believe this shit!" At 6 a.m. the next morning, it started all over again.

I knew there were a lot of people who thought I couldn't handle The Citadel. And now I had fellow cadets telling me that to my face. So I never came close to quitting. But there were at least two or three who left the very first day. These were football players, mind you, guys who were used to an above-average level of abuse, and *they* couldn't handle it. It's one thing for that many to drop out of the general population, but these were football players who had been recruited to play college football. In all, out of my entire freshmen class, at least ten to twenty percent dropped out the first year.

Then there was "Hell Night." It was more ceremonial and symbolic than anything else, but it was the official introduction to the fact that the fourth-class system—signifying the hierarchy in classes—was now in effect. It was an hour-long festival of abuse of the freshmen by the upperclassmen. All the upperclassmen were expected to participate, and it didn't take a genius to realize that the odds were not in our favor. Basically, you have over one hundred upperclassmen per company and only forty freshmen. You do the math. From that point on it wasn't only the cadets with the officer rank who could abuse you—nobody was off-limits. You were fair game for *any* upperclassman cadet on campus.

Once we made it through the initiation for football players, the rest of the F-Troop freshmen joined us and together we became the F-Troop class of 1988. We were all ordered to switch rooms in order to be integrated with the rest of the freshmen cadet population. I ended up with another football player named Jason Matthews. If opposites attract, then Jason and I were a roommate match made in heaven. Jason was from North Wilkesboro, North Carolina, a small southern town in the foothills of the Blue Ridge Mountains. He loved to listen to Hank Williams Jr., Waylon Jennings, and all the good old country boys, whereas I listened to Iron Maiden, Black Sabbath, and Bob Marley. Jason played offensive center. That's the person who starts the play by snapping the ball to the quarterback. Since I played middle linebacker, this meant I was directly across the center of the opposing side. Let's just say that Jason and I bumped heads a few times in practice. But we always left it on the field and never antagonized each other about who might have had the better day. Besides, we needed to rely on each other.

So from the second day on campus through the rest of the first year, my day started at 6 a.m. I had to be what they called "blitzed" from head to toe. My shoes had to be polished to look like glass. My name tag had to be buffed. My belt had to be nice and shiny, and my buckle—the most important piece—had to be shined to perfection. My pants and shirt had to line up in what they called a "gig line." The button line of my shirt had to line up with the button and zipper line of my pants, perfectly. Shirts had to be tucked in a certain way. We had to put cardboard inside our hats to keep them perfectly formed and stiff. My hair had to be perfect and I had to be always clean-shaven. All of this had to be done before arriving downstairs for yet more procedures by 6:20 a.m.

From 6:20 a.m. until 6:45 a.m. we were braced, and locked in formation. There were two or three sophomore corporals who just the previous year went through the same hell and got the shit beat out of them. They had to have been salivating, waiting for this opportunity to dish out the same punishment to somebody else. Every morning, Monday through Friday, they inspected us. It didn't matter how perfect we were. They screamed at us at the top of their lungs from an inch away from our faces. They spit on their finger and smudged our belt buckle with it, then told us how awful it looked. They scuffed up our shoes, pulled our shirts out. They pulled on our arms while we were in formation. One guy would tell me to recite the cadet prayer. As soon I started the prayer, another guy would scream "shut up!" The second I stopped reciting the prayer, the first guy went nuts again, screaming, "Didn't I tell you to recite the prayer?" It was like that scene from *Cool Hand Luke*, when prison guards punish Luke by making him dig a hole in the yard, only to have another guard scold him for putting dirt on the yard, and making him fill the hole back up with the dirt, several times. This stuff happened every morning of every day for a year.

Now, Charleston can be very hot and muggy. But the heat is nothing compared to the bugs and no-see-ums, which eat away at your skin. For twenty minutes every morning we braced. We couldn't move a muscle without inciting the wrath of one of these guys. And we didn't dare let them smell bug spray on us. It was prohibited as it represented a sign of weakness. We stood there in formation getting eaten alive by all these bugs and we couldn't move. You just stood there and took it. As much as anything else, that was enough to drive anyone crazy. Then in February and March, yet another challenge: it would get cold, down into the 20s at 6 a.m., and we'd have to stand in freezing conditions unable to move.

When the first formation of the day was over, they'd yell, "Knobs roll out!" That meant running on the quad and falling into formation with the rest of the company. Other than those brief moments, freshmen weren't allowed to step foot on the quad. From there we were marched to breakfast at 7 a.m. We stood at attention while bracing behind our seat. Each table seated fourteen cadets, six on either side with one at each end. Upperclassmen occupied the seats on the ends. When they told us to take our seats, we could only sit on the front three inches of the chair. We had to maintain brace—yes, while sitting—throughout breakfast. The first order of business was to ask one of the upperclassmen if he wanted something to drink. Of course, everyone is called "sir." In fact, the only three acceptable responses for a knob were: "Sir. Yes, sir," "Sir. No, sir," or "Sir. No excuse, sir." Then you had to keep watching his glass and keep it filled so that it never approached being half empty. After everyone was served, and if we were lucky enough to have a decent guy heading the table, we could eat. A lot of times we never ate a thing because of all the procedural bullshit.

If we did have food on our plates, we had to first pick up the fork, scoop up the food, put the food into our mouth, put the fork down, and then chew. After swallowing, we had to follow the same routine for every bite. In the meantime, the upperclassmen were messing with you and testing you all the while. "Buoniconti, how many moves in that rifle maneuver? What's the cadet prayer? Tell us a joke and it better be funny!" It was a constant barrage and everything directed at us was screamed. I'd get three or four bites in, if I was lucky. I was always hungry. One time I was so hungry I put an entire hamburger in my mouth in one bite. When they saw that, the guy in charge of our table started screaming, "Swallow! Swallow it right now!" I tried to swallow and the hamburger became stuck. I started choking. The guy is now screaming, "Drink!" I tried but I couldn't get anything down my throat. Eventually I threw it up right back onto my plate. I picked up the soggy hamburger, and without even dusting it off, immediately took a bite because I was so hungry. I knew I would likely not have another chance to eat. My antics grossed out everyone and ended up clearing the table. Meals were rough, man.

We had to be done with breakfast by 7:30 a.m. Then we were marched back into our rooms, where we had to change out of our inspection gear and into what was called "class brass." I would take off my belt buckle and put it aside because that was used only for inspection. I wore black, glossy shoes called Coraframs—shiny, patent leather Oxford shoes that looked like cop shoes—instead of our inspection shoes. We still had to look neat, shiny, and tight at all times. Our rooms, too, had to be perfect at all times because there would be surprise inspections.

Classes started at 8 a.m. From the moment we walked out of our rooms, it was double-time. That meant bracing and running at the same time. Of course, it wasn't as easy at that. The added twist was that we could only double-time on a one brick-wide edge on one side of the hallway near the railing. We couldn't stand or walk on any other part of the floor in the hallway. When we reached the stair-way, it was another series of issues. We couldn't walk down the stairs without permission unless no one else was around. If you reached the stairs and an upperclassman was around, you had to ask him, by name, for permission to walk down those stairs. It went like this: "Mr. Johnson, sir, cadet Buoniconti requesting to drive your stairs, sir." Only after being granted permission could I then run down that stair level. If an upperclassman happened to be on the very next level of stairs, whether he was ascending or descending, the exercise would be repeated at each level.

As tedious as that may sound, in addition to all that we had to know the name of every person in the company and their rank. If you reached the stairs and didn't know the name of someone, he'd start screaming, "You don't know my name, knob? Get down on the floor!" The worst was when there were three or four guys present, and you had to know every one of their names. You had to glance very quickly to get a look at each of them because your eyes were supposed to be focused straight ahead at all times. I had to recognize each person and their rank. And, as if that weren't enough, I had to make sure I addressed the highest-ranking person first, and asked him for permission.

If we made it down the stairs, we had to do so in double-time until we made it out the gates of the battalion. Then we could walk but only on the right side of the sidewalk. In certain areas we had to walk behind the buildings. In one part of campus, we had to walk in the gutter. At no time could we look around. We were expected to keep our eyes straight ahead at all times. All this and we hadn't even been to a class yet.

Morning classes went from 8 a.m. till noon. Then it was back to the battalion, more bracing in formation, and more getting messed with just like the morning. Eventually we rolled out and marched in formation to lunch, which lasted for thirty minutes, between 12:15 to 12:45. It was the same routine as breakfast, sitting on the front three inches of the chair, being screamed at, and barely able to eat. Then we marched back to the battalion, went to classes from 1 p.m. to 3 p.m. At that point, I would head straight to football practice. But by then— physically and psychologically exhausted—I was ready to pass out.

We were sleep-deprived and hungry from our first day on campus. I tried to sleep anywhere I could get a minute or two. I'd even fall asleep at football team meetings, which were only about fifteen minutes long. The only good thing about heading off to football practice was the fact that some of the same guys who took great joy in making my life miserable every day also happened to be football players. As a rule, football players didn't abuse teammates, even the freshmen. But for a guy like me, practice drills made for great payback. And there wasn't a thing they could do about it. That's one good reason football players didn't mess with me after the first couple weeks. It didn't matter, though, because there were plenty of other guys dishing out punishments.

Even though I was tired, it was a relief to show up at the football facility at 3:15 p.m. I didn't get to relax, but it was closer to a normal life experience compared to the rest of the day. Generally, practice went to around 5:30 p.m., which left just enough time to get back to the barracks for formation. Then we marched to 6 o'clock dinner. After dinner, football players went back to the football building for another sixty to ninety minutes. During the first two weeks of my freshman year, we practiced three times a day. The night session was either a walkthrough or a meeting. Then, between 7:30 and 10:30 p.m. we had mandatory study hall. I returned to the battalion around 11 p.m. with lights-out at 11:30 p.m. That didn't mean it was time to sleep, though. I spent however much time was necessary to shine my shoes and make sure everything was perfect for the next morning. I might hit the rack by midnight. A lot of times it was 1 a.m. before I managed to put my head down. Then, five or six hours later, it started all over again.

As if the long days weren't bad enough, my Staff Sergeant, Daniel Bridges, was straight out of Central Casting. Armed with two years of pent-up frustration from The Citadel, combined with an angry streak a mile long, he was the one guy you didn't want to irritate. Of course, even though I tried to keep a low profile, there was no doubt that I stuck out like a sore thumb. Mr. Bridges was a good ol' boy, which was in sharp contrast in attitude and personality with my Miami fast-paced, big-city upbringing. I might as well have worn a target on my back. No one was singled out more than I among the knobs in F-Troop. Some upperclassmen from other battalions and divisions walked all the way across campus just to ask: "Where's that Buoniconti knob?"

Endless in-my-face screaming, countless push-ups, and other disciplinary and hazing rituals typically followed the question. These were a normal part of life as a cadet. By the second week, Mr. Bridges could see right through my bullshit. Then came the line that would be the preface of many a bad experience: "Buoniconti," Mr. Bridges would exclaim in his Southern drawl, "you're really starting to piss me off!" It was a signal of impending hell.

As part of our training, every cadet had to learn the manual of arms with our M-14 rifle. It was just like in the movies: right shoulder arms, left shoulder arms, order arms, and so forth. I was in trouble so often with Mr. Bridges that I had to do the manual of arms all by myself standing outside his room before every morning, afternoon, and evening formation. My other Staff Sergeant, Ron Villa, was much more forgiving. We shared a few similarities in that we were both originally from Massachusetts and we were Italian. We had our share of rough moments as well but, on the whole, he went out of his way to help the football players, and especially me because I needed it most. Remember, while most of the cadets could relax after class, catch up on studies, football players practiced all day and most evenings. We had little to no time to focus on our military obligations, let alone study.

Being a football player had its benefits too. But the demands were probably double compared to other students. The physical part of football was one thing. The mental aspect was another. High school football at the level we played in South Florida was highly sophisticated. Still, I had to learn a lot of new football terminology once I arrived at The Citadel. The real benefit of being a football player came later, once the season started. We didn't have to eat meals with the regular students, which meant the players had the opportunity to eat together, like human beings. We could put our elbows on the table, sit in chairs normally and, most importantly, we could eat as much as we wanted.

Through all the abuse and stress, I never saw anybody really snap. A lot of guys dropped out of school. I don't remember anyone becoming violent over the verbal abuse. One morning, though, I did go after one guy. Some upperclassmen ordered us to herd like cattle into a stairwell, forcing us to push right up against one another. This was an open stairwell that went up four stories. As soon as we piled into that small space, there were guys spitting on us from above. I went crazy. I was three-quarters up the first level before a bunch of guys were able to stop me. Everyone has limits. Getting spit on while smashed against a group of guys was mine.

On the field, things were different. As it turned out, I was one of only two freshmen to letter and make the traveling team. On Day 1, I made a point of getting noticed. I knew coaches were probably concerned with my size. I lost ten to fifteen pounds those first two weeks. Just to make sure they didn't let size confuse their judgment, I did two things in the first scrimmage. First, I blitzed on almost every play. Second, I drilled the quarterback even though he was wearing a red jersey, which meant he couldn't be hit. I didn't care. I wanted to be noticed, and I unloaded on him. I started the first week at fourth team middle linebacker. When the first week of hitting ended, I was second team.

I played in every game that season, all on special teams. I was on the kickoff and punt return teams. On the kickoff team I was what we called the "maniac," the wedge buster. My job was to run downfield as fast as I could and lay my body out to destroy the wedge of blockers trying to protect the kick returner. So many players in college and in professional football have been hurt attempting the same thing, that a wedge of blockers on the kickoff return is now illegal. On the punt return team I led the return wall.

I learned a lot of football at The Citadel, particularly in terms of technique. In high school I played on instinct. In college I learned blocking schemes, which made my freshman season a valuable learning year. By the end of the season I knew how to avoid blocks and read plays. To that point in my football life I never talked much football with my dad. But as I started to grasp the nuances of the game, I talked with him more about various techniques. I even remember throwing around a football with him, something I never did when I was younger.

We had a pretty good team my freshman year. We lost to Furman for the Southern Conference Championship and finished 7-4, with two of those losses to the much larger schools, Georgia Tech and South Carolina.

Everything went well on the football field. Not so much in the classroom. I had a 1.6 grade-point-average after my first semester, passing all my classes with Cs and Ds. Given all the stress put on freshmen, it was an accomplishment. I wasn't a very good student to begin with. I was nearly kicked out of school over an accusation made by another student. I was accused of cheating on a test—an honor code violation—that, as you can imagine, is a high offense at a military institution. If anyone had bothered to look at my test score, they would have realized I didn't cheat. I finished my test, and I was walking to the front of the class to hand it in. I asked the guy next to me, who had also finished his test, "What did you say on the essay?" The guy freaked out. At The Citadel the code of honor is taken seriously. A cadet "cannot lie, cheat or steal, nor tolerate those who do." If a cadet sees anyone violate one of those and he doesn't report the person, then the witness is considered equally guilty. The guy felt compelled to turn me in. The fact that I had turned in my paper apparently didn't matter. He said I asked him a question about something that was on the test, which technically was true. But there was no possible benefit to me.

As a result, I had to go through The Citadel Honor Court, a trip not many survive. The process is as thorough as any legal proceeding anywhere in the country. The Honor Court is made up of senior cadets, who act as jury. Their decision is final. I had to give a deposition to the cadet prosecuting attorney. I had my own legal team, the F-Troop Honor Court legal representative, Daniel Stubley, my friend and senior teammate Jim Gabrish, and his friend who agreed to be our lead counsel, Chris Clark, the Regimental XO (Executive Officer). Chris was the second highest command in the school. Jim served as intimidator and interrogator. I knew I was innocent, but I worried I could still be had on a technicality.

On the legal side the deck was stacked in my favor. I still had to testify. My coach even had to testify. There were character witnesses, cross-examinations, and everything else you would see in a regular trial. When the trial ended, I climbed onto the rooftop looking out over the campus. It was January of my freshman year. After all the abuse, after an otherwise successful start to my college life, all I could think about was whether I was going to be sent home later that day.

My legal team turned out to be as persuasive outside of court as it was during the court proceedings. Oddly enough, one of the witnesses couldn't remember exactly what he had heard. I was found not guilty.

About two weeks later I needed an emergency appendectomy. I honestly think it was a result of all the stress around the trial. Sadly, but to further put life as a Citadel freshman in perspective, emergency surgery was one of my better experiences that year.

The attack came on during the early morning hours of a Monday. At first, I thought it was from all the drinking I had done the night before. Then, as the pain worsened, I realized something was wrong. I stumbled out of my room, down the stairs, and out of the barracks. The infirmary was about a quarter of a mile away. It was freezing outside. By the time I got there I was crawling. I made it all the way to the front steps and managed to push the button to alert the nurse on duty. She opened the door, let me crawl in, and then said, "You're supposed to call first." As I felt myself about to die (at least I felt that way), she said, "The doctor doesn't get here for a couple more hours." By 8 a.m. I was rushed to the emergency room of the Medical University of South Carolina, then directly to surgery.

My mother arrived at the hospital wearing a mink coat. She had come directly from President Ronald Reagan's inauguration in Washington, DC.

After surgery I remained in the hospital for a few days before being transferred to the infirmary back on campus. The doctor told me to stay in the infirmary as long as necessary. I did exactly as he prescribed. I milked it for an entire month—sleeping and eating to my heart's content. I had to get up and go to class. Then I'd head right back to the infirmary. At first I had so much swelling that I couldn't even button my pants. After three or four weeks of the general's wife bringing in fresh-baked cookies, I was just fat. I had to go to The Cadet Store and buy new pants. Around the four-week mark I started to feel guilty. I knew the abuse the rest of my classmates were enduring, so I voluntarily returned to the routine.

Due to surgery-related school absences, as well as my usual lackadaisical attitude toward studying, I was put on academic probation. Alone, that wasn't too bad. I also was on military probation for the many run-ins with Mr. Bridges and other upperclassmen. Both probations had me restricted to campus, in some cases restricted to my room, and in the extreme cases, marching hours on end as punishment.

Starting to sound familiar? It was like reliving a nightmare. I thought college was supposed to be fun. I was back in the same routine as high school.

Anyone who wasn't on academic and military restrictions could leave campus. I was on both lists, which meant I was officially confined; committed was more like it. That didn't stop me completely, though. I'd get somebody to sleep in my bed on Saturday nights so I could stay out all night with the guys or a girlfriend. Come on, I followed *most* of the rules. You didn't think those would stop me? I was careful, but I was managing to have it my way.

My dad was still working for U.S. Tobacco. Every week a care package arrived with three or four rolls of chewing tobacco. I used them for bribes. There were a lot of Southern boys at The Citadel who enjoyed a good dip. Between the dip and my mom's care packages, I used everything I could to bribe my commanding officer, Glenn Shull, and executive officer, Max Kuhns, to look the other way once in a while. I'd give each of them five cans of Skoal® or Copenhagen®. Believe me, it made a difference. There was one store on campus and the smokeless tobacco would be sold out within twenty minutes of being restocked. That made me the only game in town when it came to smokeless tobacco. My mom sent me care packages every two weeks. We're not talking chips and cookies. She sent Italian sausage, salami, pepperoni, cheese, and crackers. Everyone knew when the packages arrived because they could smell the food.

I used every asset to con favors. All the scamming I did in high school proved to be a great training ground for The Citadel. And I needed every trick and con I could come up with. You know how they say some people go to jail and learn how to be an even better, or worse criminal (depending on how you define "ability")? Well, I learned how to be sneaky, conniving, and AWOL (Absent Without Official Leave) without being caught. I found every hole in the fence. I had to be extremely careful and cunning. Military-trained cadets were the guards. But getting past my mom since childhood prepared me well.

Once I was on double probation, the stakes were as high as they could get. If I got caught, it meant immediate dismissal. No second chances. No "Pass Go and Collect $200" and definitely no "Get Out of Jail Free" card. A cadet could be sent home, no questions asked. I didn't care. I was very careful. It was the only way I retained a sense of self.

As May approached, so did the light at the end of the tunnel. On the last day of school before graduation, all freshmen were subjected to one more hour of abuse and torture called "Hell Night," an homage to our final duty as freshmen. That last hour, believe it or not, was every bit as bad, or worse, than any episode I faced throughout the year.

In the end, all of the freshmen F-Troopers gathered in a circle and did eighty-eight push-ups in honor of our class. Then, as quickly as it started eight months earlier, the abuse was over. We lined up for one last time. Every upperclassman in F-Troop shook our hands in recognition of completing our freshman year.

Chapter 13

Swamp Man

I made it through my freshman year. Everyone in the Buoniconti household was ecstatic. But I couldn't go home right away. I had to stay at The Citadel for the entire summer of 1985 to attend both sessions of summer school. That was to give me a chance to qualify academically for another year of college.

In the summer, life around campus was relaxed, more like a kid going to a regular college. I could go to class in shorts and a T-shirt. There was no marching or anything like that. Since I was now "recognized" and no longer a freshman, the abuse was dialed way back, and pretty much nonexistent during the summer.

During the first summer session I lived in the barracks. I went to class every day. It was my first taste of a normal college experience because the nightlife was great. I had fun, but I also focused on working out. I wanted to get bigger and stronger by the time August rolled around. It was a reasonable expectation because I was only eighteen years old heading into my sophomore year. Still, that was the least of my concerns.

When the second summer session started, I left the barracks and moved into an off-campus apartment with a friend. My parents weren't happy with the decision because they knew there would be even more distractions with not even a nominal amount of oversight. They were right, of course. I had two run-ins with the police, the second resulting in me being arrested for shoplifting and resisting arrest.

The two of us were caught trying to steal steaks from a local grocery store, a stupid idea we came up with after some drinking. I slid a steak into my pants, and then walked out the front door. I was out by the car waiting for my friend when I looked back. He was being escorted out in handcuffs. I decided to start walking in hopes of escaping the scene of the crime. When I finally turned around there were five people heading toward me. My first instinct was to run.

The chase lasted three hours. Eventually the police brought in dogs and even a helicopter. I ran through swamps, trees, and brush, all of which produced deep scratches and gouges up and down my arms and legs. I finally made it back to the house. I was covered head to toe in mud, blood, sweat, and the stinking smell of swamp water. My buddy took one look at me and said, "Oh my god. They know. They know who you are. They're going to come to practice tomorrow and drag you off the field in cuffs."

I had previous experience with the local police, one detective in particular. He caught a friend and me smoking weed earlier that summer. He didn't arrest us, but the incident would come back to haunt me. I called the police station and asked for the detective. He came on the line and said, "Oh my god, are you in trouble! The best thing you can do is come down here right now and turn yourself in. Get here fast, while I'm still on duty. There are twenty guys in this place who want to kick your ass for dragging them through the swamps for three hours."

I had been in swamps up to my neck. I didn't have time to think about the snakes, alligators, and associated dangers. I was more worried about the dogs chasing me from behind. I took a shower and headed down to the police department. Later on, I was told there were nine officers, the dogs, and a helicopter looking for me. The fact I still got away really pissed them off. I was released on bond, but I never told my parents. The bond was only one hundred dollars. Why didn't we use that money to buy some food? I guess it was easier raising cash from friends when you need to get out of jail compared to needing a meal. The cops did me a favor too. They pleaded the charge down to a secondary misdemeanor. All I got was six months probation.

Needless to say, I had a little trouble getting through the summer. Somehow, though, I scraped by and qualified for my sophomore year. Not without more drama, however. Two weeks before the season started, I was at football practice when the head coach called me into his office. I walked into the room and he said, "I know you're doing drugs and I know you're dealing drugs." I put two and two together and realized one of the cops told somebody about my summer exploits, particularly the pot smoking incident. The information was relayed to my coach. I certainly wasn't dealing drugs. I wasn't doing drugs either, except for smoking a little pot here and there. My coach didn't believe me.

"You can do one of two things," he said. "You can take a drug test, or you can go home."

I told him I'd take a drug test right then and there. Who was I kidding? I probably had just smoked the night before. As usual, I needed to come up with an escape plan. I went directly from his office to the locker room.

I went from teammate to teammate with one question: "When's the last time you smoked pot or did drugs?" I couldn't find anybody who could pass a test any better than I could. Luckily, I ran into one guy who said, "Well, I haven't smoked in about three weeks. But I've been drinking a lot of pickle juice." I'm thinking, "Does drinking pickle juice clean the pot out of your system?" I had no other choice. I bet my entire college career on a guy drinking pickle juice. I bagged up his urine, tucked the bag into my pants and headed over to the infirmary. There was a doctor waiting for me with cup in hand when I arrived. I walked into the bathroom. The doctor peered over my shoulder through the entire process. I approached the urinal and told the doctor, "I can't go with someone looking over my shoulder. You're giving me stage fright." He walked back a few steps and stood just outside the door, which he kept open. As calmly as possible, I tore a small hole in the bag and squeezed the contents into the cup. I finished, pushed the bag back into my shorts, walked out, and handed him the specimen.

Of course, I was scared to death until the results came back two weeks later. I couldn't concentrate on anything. The first two weeks of my sophomore season were a blur. I didn't focus on school. I wasn't focused on football, either. And it showed. I should have beaten out a senior for the starting middle linebacker spot, but I wasn't all there. To be honest, he was playing better than me. Finally, in the week leading up to our first game, the results came back. I headed back into the head coach's office.

"The results are negative," he said. "OK, I'm glad to see that. I just wanted to make sure that if you miss a tackle it's because of talent and not because you're on drugs."

I said, "Coach, you should know by now that I don't miss tackles."

From that moment on I started teeing off on people in practice and especially in games. My head was clear. The stress was gone. It was like a new lease on life. I was taking advantage of every moment. My head was 100 percent in the game. It was like getting an adrenaline rush that didn't wear off. I was finally free to just play football. For the coaches and my teammates, it was as if a switch had been flipped. By the second week, I was playing as well, if not better, than the starting linebacker, Richard Brock. Richard was a great guy, very humble and always cordial despite the fact that I was breathing down his neck. It didn't matter whether it was practice or games, I was making a statement and everyone knew it. Richard was still playing the majority of the minutes, but when I was on the field I played well.

At one point I went to my coach and said, "Coach, don't you believe that the best player should start?"

He knew what I was talking about.

"I know the scheme better than Richard does and I should start. If I'm not going to play here, then I'll leave and go play somewhere else."

I had started making inquiries about transferring to Florida State, then walking onto the football team. It was the same feeling I experienced as a freshman in high school. I was a better player than the guy ahead of me, and I couldn't stand what I felt was the unfairness of it all.

I knew I could play at the college level. Despite a summer of distractions, I reported for practice weighing a solid 220 pounds. I was almost exactly the size my father was when he played in the NFL, yet I was still eighteen years old a month into the season.

My coach knew how good I could be. He heard the rumors about other schools. He tried to talk me out of leaving. I needed to be on the field. It was one thing to watch and learn as a freshman. I'd had enough of that. The coach played me a little more often, but I was done standing on the sidelines.

When I was in high school Hall of Fame, NFL coach Don Shula told my dad, "Marc has the ability to play professional football." I always thought I could play in the NFL, at least as a special teams player. To this day, I watch games and I know that I had the ability, intellect, determination, and general craziness to be a professional football player. I might have been a special teams player, but I could have survived and even thrived at that level.

After talent, attitude and toughness distinguish players who play in the NFL; a player has to be able to flip a switch and get to another level on the field. Off the field I was a fun-loving guy. On game day I turned into somebody else. It was a little like Dr. Jekyll and Mr. Hyde. I never really talked about that aspect of the game with my father. We talked more about the intricacies of football as I got older, like the ability to be in the right place at the right time by knowing how to read tendencies. Like my dad, I got by on the field by using my knowledge of the game. I had average size, but I knew how to hit. I knew how to get into position quickly to make that hit. That's how my dad thrived in the NFL. I probably had a little more quickness than either my dad or my brother. My brother ran 4.6 or 4.7 seconds in the forty-yard dash. I was able to get down to 4.4 consistently and, once in a while, a little below that. All of us were tough enough. My dad lasted fifteen seasons despite being considered too small. Nicky played his freshman year at Duke with a broken thumb and a knee injury. He had surgery on both shoulders and still came back and played.

At the time, I never thought about getting drafted. I just knew I could play at the next level. It was becoming a reasonable expectation, or at least I thought it was. I felt as though I was in a good position, either way. My dad was president of U.S. Tobacco, living in Connecticut. If I had the ability to play professional football, great, that was my number one choice. If that didn't work out, then maybe I'd get into the tobacco business and work for my dad. What could be better than working with your father? I thought it all the way through. If I stayed in school and graduated from The Citadel, then I would always have the option of going into the Air Force. At The Citadel you could choose which branch of the military you wanted to join—Army, Navy, Marines, Air Force, or Coast Guard. By my junior year I had to make a decision one way or another. Or I could choose to bypass the military altogether. I picked the Air Force right away. If I made it through, then I'd graduate as an officer, a second lieutenant. I had a taste of military life at The Citadel. It was something I could deal with.

Then, as if on cue, fate intervened. Richard tore up his knee in our fourth game, against Marshall. The position was open and it was all mine. I didn't put the idea of leaving The Citadel completely out of my mind, but I was ready for what came next. As the proverb says, "Be careful what you wish for."

On the Monday following the Marshall game, I brought a whole new level of intensity to practice. As the starting linebacker, I was in charge of the huddle and the focal point of the defense. Off the field, I was the new media angle for the local sports writers, which brought a refreshed feeling of arrogance. My ego ate it all up. After practice I walked through the training room. I noticed a kind of neck roll that I had never seen before. Some football players use a neck roll that is attached to the shoulder pads like a horseshoe that is intended to support the back and sides of the neck. I wore a neck roll starting in high school, and the one I was using at The Citadel was simply a rolled-up hand towel that had been inserted into a thin sheath, nothing fancy. This new neck roll was different. It was cool looking. It had a skinnier roll with a thick attachment in the middle of the back for extra support. I remember thinking to myself, "Wow, now this looks badass!"

Even though I was a lot like my father and brother in many respects, vanity was never something that entered their minds. It did with me. While the three of us played the game with equal intensity and preparation, I was the only one who wanted to make sure that I looked good doing it. So when I made the seemingly insignificant decision to change my neck roll from the tried-and-true one to the fancier and cooler one, it started a chain of events with a ripple effect that would exceed the reaches of my imagination. Only in time do we come to understand the significance of one decision or another. As I've said, it's not just the choices we make, but it's the ones we fail to make as well.

At practice the next day I was covering a receiver during a scrimmage. When he attempted to make a catch, I hit him hard, as usual, and jarred the ball loose for an incomplete pass. But I got the worst of it. As I made the tackle, my neck was bent backwards. I had the sudden sensation of a "stinger." A stinger is a common physical sensation. After contact, a burning, numbing sensation radiates from the base of your neck and down your arm. I hadn't had a stinger since high school. While the feeling usually dissipates after a few minutes, once a player gets a stinger, he's more susceptible to another one. Who was I kidding? I was just about to start my first college football game. I wasn't going to let a few stingers keep me off the field.

My first start came against the Virginia Military Institute (VMI) in Lexington, Virginia. About an hour before the game, after getting taped up, I walked outside and sat next to the locker room door, which was beneath the stadium. I looked up and there was my dad. I had no idea he was coming. I couldn't believe it. I stood up and gave him a big hug. It was so meaningful to me that my father would go to the trouble of driving hours out of his way just to see his son make his first start.

My brother's team, Duke, was playing at the University of Virginia that day, so my dad came down to see me start my first college game. Then at halftime he jumped back in his car and drove to see the second half of Nicky's game.

I'm sure he was proud of us. Nicky became the starting middle linebacker at Duke in his sophomore season too. The next week we played in Charleston. We recorded the first Citadel shutout in ten years, and my parents and sister Gina were there to see it all. It was a great weekend. I remember my father being happy. Not only was I starting and playing really well, I was in school. All three of us were in college, my dad's career was going great, and we were together.

For my parents, I'm sure they felt life couldn't get much better.

Chapter 14

Boys to Men

DAD: I made life miserable for a lot of quarterbacks. That's what middle linebackers are supposed to do. If a middle linebacker is really effective, then the moment the quarterback steps up to the center he has to be aware of where that middle linebacker is at all times. The quarterback had to account for me. If he didn't have to account for the opposing middle linebacker, then that linebacker shouldn't even be on the field. He's not having an impact on what's going on.

That's why when I'm asked who is the greatest middle linebacker to ever play, in a nanosecond I say Dick Butkus. Why Butkus? Why not Jack Lambert? Why not Willie Lanier? Why not Ray Nitschke? When Dick Butkus was in his position the first thing that opposing quarterback wanted to know was where Butkus was and who was going to block him. Left unattended, he was just such a force. He made quarterbacks change plays because of where he was.

I played in the golden era. In the history of the game there will never be that many superior linebackers playing at the same time. It really became unfair to them because when it came to choosing the All-Pro team, there were so many great middle linebackers. Just because you weren't picked didn't mean you weren't great. Lee Roy Jordan in Dallas, Tommy Nobis in

Atlanta, Mike Curtis in Baltimore. Butkus, Nitschke, Lanier, Lambert, and myself were their contemporaries too.

In the history of the National Football League, Jack Ham and I hold the career record for interceptions by a middle linebacker with 32. That's a little-known statistic. The point is, that there are a lot of things that go into a player making it into the Hall of the Fame. It took me a little while, but I think there are guys who have been left out of the mix who deserve to be in.

By the time Nicky and Marc started to play and have success, their high school stadiums were sold out. It was a lot of fun. Michael Shula, Don's son, was the starting quarterback for Columbus in Marc's junior year. Don and I would go to the games. We never could sit next to each other because we were so critical. As a matter of fact, I couldn't even watch the game sitting next to Marc's mom. I would see things that were so basic to me that, when they didn't go right, it was hard to watch. I would sit away from Terry, and Don would sit away from me.

Early on I made a deal with myself. I would never interfere with Marc or Nicky even when they played at the Pop Warner level. I never coached them, and I never got involved. I thought it would be unfair to the other kids in the league if a professional player helped one team when the opposing team was being coached by a father just trying to help out. I don't know whether it would have turned out to be an advantage or not, but I made up my mind that I wasn't going to interfere with the coaches. I did coach my boy's baseball teams, and I coached my daughter's softball team.

Marc and I never really talked a whole lot about football. I did talk to Nicky quite a bit because he was willing to listen. By the time Marc got home, it was a lot later than when Nicky got home. Nicky and I used to sit down on the couch and talk about the game. I never told him what he did wrong unless he asked me. I never commented on what he did right either, unless he asked me for my opinion.

They were totally different kinds of players. Nicky was early to practice whether it was baseball or football and the last one to leave the field. He was working 100 percent of the time. He loved playing linebacker. He was a ferocious hitter for his size. You could count on him to be there every single game and to make the plays. Marc, on the other hand, had more natural ability, but Marc would be the last one to practice and the first one off the field. He would freelance more than anybody on the team. He would do what he thought was the right thing whether it was what the coach wanted him to do. Marc could get away with it because he had phenomenal natural ability. He was fast. He could hit. He was an offense's worst nightmare.

In terms of style, they couldn't have been more different. They each got the job done but in a different way. When Nicky was a freshman at Duke he made seventeen tackles against Georgia Tech in his first start. He was ACC Defensive Player of the Week in the first game he ever started in college. Marc had the natural ability to go further than The Citadel. I think Marc would have been a 220- to 225-pound linebacker by the time he graduated, and he would have been given the opportunity to try out for the pros.

I would say that I was more like Nicky than Marc in many ways. I was always on time. I was always studying. I was always disciplined. But I also had Marc's athletic ability, which was a good combination to have— Nicky's dependability and Marc's speed and quickness.

We'll obviously never know how far Marc could have gone, but Don Shula said Marc was one of the best linebackers he had ever seen.

Chapter 15

A Little Brother Grows Up

GINA: Once Marc got to The Citadel we became even closer. I went up from Gainesville to Charleston to see him in September of his sophomore year along with my parents. It was great to see Marc play. I remember him being so proud. After all the trouble growing up, here he was becoming a young man. He was in college. He was starting on the football team. Everyone was proud.

There's a lot of prestige that goes with The Citadel in Charleston. It seemed to me that he was working things out. I knew he was always going to be a wild man. Was I worried? A little bit. I wasn't fearful that something awful was going to happen to him, though. I was just so proud of him. He seemed so much more mature and grown up.

Marc was a tough kid. He had amazing survival skills. He learned some of them from getting beat up all the time by his older brother. But Marc was tough. He could deal with The Citadel. Unless you have experienced that level of discipline, it's hard to even imagine what Marc went through day to day.

You never would have known it was anything more than your basic college experience by looking at Marc, though. He never complained. For a kid who had struggled through every grade in school, it was wonderful to see how proud he was of himself. He had always been good on the football field, and he was on that day too.

The one thing I noticed at dinner following the game, though, was that Marc's neck was sore. He couldn't turn his neck from side to side to have a conversation. He had to turn his whole body toward the person talking. I told him, "Marc, you've got to take care of your neck. What's going on with it anyway?"

This was two weeks before I got "The Call." It was clear he had a problem. Still, they let him play. He was just a kid. Of course Marc was going to play if they allowed him onto the field. It was not in Marc's nature to stay on the sidelines if the coaches said he could play.

Chapter 16

A Pain in the Neck

By the time I started my first college game my neck was sore. From the moment I got my first college "stinger," every time I made a really good hit I felt a variation of the same sensation. By the time we played Virginia Military Institute (VMI, or what we jokingly referred to them as "Virginia's Marching Idiots"), I was sore to the point of being conscious of the pain. I remember one play when the ball carrier was in front of me. Normally I would have unloaded on him. I had the presence of mind to think about the pain that would follow if I had hit him squarely with my entire upper body. It would have hurt me a lot more than him. My parents didn't know about my injury. This was football at The Citadel. Being a military school, there already was a premium on toughness. When you layer the football mentality over the prevailing culture of the institution, aches and pains become just part of the game. Move on, or move off the field.

In the beginning, I really didn't question whether or not I could continue to play. My neck hurt, but a lot of things hurt when you play college football. There is always a level of discomfort for anyone who played as much and as hard as I did. You deal with it. That was my thought process. But after the VMI game, my neck really started to bother me. I began receiving therapy in the training room, but the pain was intense.

I played the next week at home against Davidson College. After that game, however, the pain went to a new level. My father noticed something was wrong just in watching me play. My neck had only a very slight range of motion. I could barely move my head side to side.

Aside from the pain, it was another great weekend. My mom, dad, and my sister came into Charleston to see the game. At dinner that night, my dad made a point of telling me to get my neck checked out. He was very clear about wanting me to see a doctor.

Initially, I went into the trainer's room once a day for heat, ice, and massage treatments. After the Davidson game, I was in the trainer's room twice a day for treatments. The following week we played the University of Tennessee at Chattanooga on the road. On the first play of the game, the quarterback took off on a bootleg. He never saw me coming. Just as he cut back right in front of me I hit him as hard as I could. Normally I would have taken his head off. This time I got the worst of it. The pain shot through my neck and down into my arms with a new level of intensity. From that play forward, I played the game without moving my neck as much as possible. I tackled with my shoulder diving at their legs. I could not hit anybody face up like I normally would. I knew I'd end up on the wrong side of the pain. And it was intense.

I played the entire game. I made twelve or fifteen tackles, had an interception, blocked a field goal, and recovered a fumble. I was named the Southern Conference "Defensive Player of the Week" despite playing with no neck! I nearly scored a touchdown too. I ran fifty yards with an interception. I was so out of gas at the end that I had to dive for the end zone. I came up a yard short. Still, I dreaded every play of that game because of the pain. Every hit produced another shock throughout my upper body. Each one seemed more intense than the one before.

I brought a hammock along and rigged it up in the back of the bus. I thought the hammock would ease the pain I felt when sitting in a regular seat. I used the hammock on the way to the game. On the bus ride back from Chattanooga, the bouncing up and down was intolerable. After that game, I lay in the hammock with ice around my neck. I literally cried all the way back to Charleston. Everyone recog nized that I was in severe pain, including the coaches and trainer. We were probably on that bus for six or seven hours. It was unbearable. At that point, I started to become concerned. Now it was just constant neck pain.

I spoke to my dad that Sunday. I told him my neck had become much worse. He was concerned enough that he called the coach and told him to get me in for an X-ray. The following week I wore a "red jersey" which meant I was not to have any contact whatsoever in practice. The progression from comfort to intense pain went like this: After the VMI game I wore a yellow jersey, which meant limited contact in practice. After the Tennessee game, I wore a red jersey. No contact. On Monday morning following the ride back from Tennessee, I was diagnosed with a sprained neck, with 75 percent motion restriction. That entire week I was in the trainer's room three times a day. On Wednesday I walked out of a meeting room and the coaches were talking. They came up to me and said, "Can you play?" I told them I didn't know whether I could. They told me they needed an answer one way or another. The tone was clear: you need to play. Still, I kept telling them that I just didn't know.

The pain was constant to the point that I couldn't even use a pillow to sleep. The pain associated with arching my neck to accommodate the depth of the pillow was intolerable. Midweek I met with the trainer. That's when he and I started discussing a way of alleviating the pain that I was experiencing every time I moved my head backwards. I was after a solution that would prevent my neck from jostling. Our conversation resulted in the manufacture of a makeshift contraption designed to keep my head in place. The rationale, which seems ridiculous in retrospect, was that if I had something that limited the movement of my neck then I would be able to tolerate the pain enough to play.

"Let's build a big collar on the back of your neck so that it can't snap back" the trainer said. We took a hard rubber collar—a kind I hadn't used before—and built it up by adding several layers of padding cut into strip shapes. Then he made a recommendation: "To make sure your head won't move, we'll attach a strap from the front of your helmet to your shoulder pads." He fitted the apparatus on me. At that point I wasn't able to move my head back at all. At the same time the immobility caused by the contraption made it impossible for me to lift my head so that I wasn't able to look up—something I would have to do to read the plays, look for oncoming blockers, cover players, and make tackles. It made me completely vulnerable, to say the least. At the time I weighed any skepticism against the alternative: pain. Weeks later I was told that when my teammate Scott Thompson saw the con-traption he said, "Marc's going to break his fucking neck."

By the time Saturday rolled around my neck felt a little better. I didn't practice all week. I was getting therapy sessions constantly. I also wore a soft collar, the kind people wear for whiplash. What I didn't know at the time was that wearing the soft collar probably did more harm than good. The muscles in my neck were atrophying from lack of use.

At that point I was barely getting by in school. I couldn't complain, though. I might have been on the verge of serious academic trouble, but my neck was the only real problem in my life. Honestly, I think I had a good chance of flunking out of school. But when you're a starter on the football team and you're kicking ass like I was, then it's a whole different world. I was profiled on *The Tom Moore Show*, our head coach's television program. They showed highlights of me making the plays that earned me conference defensive player of the week. I was also an upperclassman, so things around school had improved dramatically.

With the exception of my poor academic outlook and the pain in my neck, life wasn't all that bad.

Chapter 17

Whose Arm Is That Again?

In the week heading into the East Tennessee State game, our team focused on a junior running back named Herman Jacobs. Our coaches watched him on film. The fact that San Francisco was scouting him had trickled down the grapevine and into our locker room. All week we had a player on the "scout" team wearing Herman's number. He was the one guy we had to contain.

What I didn't know was that East Tennessee had a player wearing a jersey with my name and number. They were as concerned about keeping me from disrupting their offense as we were about keeping Herman from exploiting our defense. What they didn't know was that I had no contact in practice all week.

The closer we came to game time, the more I wanted to play. I wanted nothing more than to be on the field. I knew the coaches wanted me to play. The way I looked at it was, "Yeah, my neck hurts, but not as badly as it did seven days earlier." By the time we got to the stadium, or "mini-dome" as it was called, my mind was locked into game mode.

The psychological sensation was familiar. Every time I prepared to play, whether in a game, practice, pick-up basketball, or Frisbee with my friends, I felt the same rush. Whatever it was that began to stir is difficult to describe—energy, excited anxiety, exuberance, nervousness—all woven into a whirlwind of emotions and thoughts. It's the veritable Jekyll to Hyde transformation. I was more intensely focused on everything in front of me. I became hyper-vigilant and even more centered in the moment. The excitement was simply overwhelming. When it came down to it, the selfless desire to play for my team easily outweighed what would have been a selfish decision to safeguard my well-being. I thought: "I guess I'm going to have a sore neck all week again. I can deal with that."

I never gave it another thought from that moment on. Once I was on the field the adrenaline took over. The first series was no big deal, three and out. We got the ball back and marched down the field for a 7-0 lead. I don't recall feeling pain. What I do remember is feeling my movement restricted. At one point I tried looking up into the stands but my helmet rode down on my eyebrows. I realized that on a pass play I probably wasn't going to be able to see the ball.

On first down after the kickoff, Herman ran straight up the middle for a nine-yard gain. I was chop-blocked at the knees and never had a chance. They got me on that one. On second down with a yard to go, they ran the same play. This time it was Herman and me, one on one. Denied! I hit him good and hard, stopping him cold for no gain.

Now it was third down and a yard to go for a first down. He won the first one. I won the second. It all came down to a single play. This time it was an option play going to my left. The quarterback rolled out with Herman behind him. The center tried to cut me, but I fought off the block. The ball was pitched to Herman, who quickly tried to head up field and get the one yard he needed.

I was scraping to the outside when I saw Herman cut up the field. My teammate and outside linebacker, Joel Thompson, dove at Herman's feet and tripped him up. It sent Herman flying through the air. I was running as hard and fast as I could. How was I going to make the tackle? Any way I could. By the time I got to Herman, he was upside down, his feet in the air, one hand reaching for the first down but still lunging forward as if about to do a cartwheel.

I took off and dove straight at him. I wanted to hit Herman as hard as I could to slow his momentum and prevent the first down. All I needed was to get a piece of him.

They say that whenever you make plans, God laughs. He had to have been hysterical as I plotted my future early in my sophomore year of college. I had big plans. It somehow seems reasonable that the way I got hurt was wholly consistent with the way I had been going through life. I hurtled myself through the air toward Herman without knowing the precise consequences—without a destination. I didn't know where I'd hit him because both of us were flying. That's pretty much how I had been living my life. I never planned to be at The Citadel. I had never even heard of the place when one of their coaches first came to recruit me. I had no plans, no direction. I didn't know where I'd end up. So, I landed in Charleston, South Carolina.

Yet, in that moment I had a plan. I knew exactly where I was going. I might have been flying with reckless abandon with a sore neck, but I was focused on the task at hand.

The next thing I knew there was contact. I felt nothing. I fell to the turf and the momentum rolled me onto my right side at an awkward angle. I saw an arm drop to the ground. I remember wondering whose arm it was because the arm seemed out of place amid the tangle of bodies. The next sensation I felt was numbness. Then I struggled to breathe.

Right away I knew. I don't know how I knew, but I knew. The arm that flopped onto the ground, as if it had been detached from somebody's body, was mine. I always knew that third-and-one was a game-changing moment. But I had no way of knowing it would be a life-changing moment.

I was paralyzed.

Chapter 18

The Call: College Park

NICK JR: All kids want to be like their dad, right? Marc and I played football from the moment we could start playing. Marc cared about certain things, but in general he had a very cavalier outlook on life. I was a bit of a hard-ass when it came to Marc just like any other older brother.

I ended up going to Duke on a full-ride scholarship even though I was barely five-foot-ten and 190 pounds. I knew Marc was good enough to play college football. The academic requirements weren't exactly stringent in those days. Even though he was kind of a delinquent, a lot of the teachers liked him because he had such a good personality. For the most part he was making the kind of bad decisions kids do when they are young. But Marc was a very likable guy, and most people felt that way about him. He was charming, and he certainly wasn't stupid. Marc was every bit as smart, if not smarter, than Gina and me, but he didn't care.

All I knew about The Citadel was that it was close to Durham, North Carolina, where I was at Duke. I thought the military environment would be good for Marc. I also never thought he'd make it through. I didn't think he would ever put up with all the crap freshmen had to endure. But I was proud of him. He looked awesome in his uniform. He seemed like a different kid until I realized later on that he really wasn't much different than he had been in high school. He ran with a crowd at The Citadel that was every bit as wild as his buddies back in Miami.

Our grandfather gave me an old beat-up car to use at Duke. I drove it over to The Citadel to drop it off for Marc the summer between his freshman and sophomore year. Marc wasn't supposed to leave campus, though that never stopped him. He covered himself up with blankets and lay on the floorboards in the backseat. He told me, "Just keep driving when you hit the gate. They won't stop you." That's how we got out on the town. He had no fear.

That was a rare time for us in college because we were busy with school and football most of the time. We didn't communicate that much because Marc wasn't allowed to have a phone his first year at The Citadel. I wasn't able to see him play in college, either. I'm not sure he saw me play in college other than a game or two that might have been on television. Later on I saw some tape of Marc playing at The Citadel. He was a free spirit, a great athlete. He was a smart, tough player, with a linebacker's mentality. I wish I had been able to see him play more.

The day I received the call we were playing at the University of Maryland. Apparently, the public address announcer had been paging my parents during the game because somebody from Duke thought they were at the game in College Park. I never heard any of this down on the field. It wasn't something I would have been listening for anyway. Maryland beat us pretty good that day and, as a player, I was pissed off after the game. I'm sure the coaches didn't say anything nice given the result. I showered and life seemed normal.

I was getting dressed when my head coach, Steve Sloan, came over.

"Your brother was hurt in a game today against East Tennessee State in Johnson City. You probably need to call someone to make sure everything is OK."

I thought to myself, "I'm not going to worry about it. I'm sure it's no big deal." At the time, I didn't realize that my coach knew the urgency of the situation. He didn't feel comfortable giving me the grim details in front of the whole team, which I appreciated.

"I'm sure I'll catch up with him tomorrow," I said.

"No, no. Your brother was hurt badly. You need to call your family."

I was used to my own injuries, and seeing my dad hurt when he was playing. By that point, I had experienced my share of injuries at Duke. I thought, "How bad could it be?"

Then I was led out of the locker room and around the stadium to the press box. I was told, "You are going to be met there." As I walked I knew something bad had occurred. Somebody from the athletic director's office at the University of Maryland took me around through a tunnel. He handed me a phone and said, "You need to talk to this person."

It was a doctor from Johnson City. I picked up, and told him who I was.

"Your brother has been hurt."

"OK, well, tell me straight up. What's the problem?"

"He's paralyzed. He's never going to walk again."

That's literally what he said. I was the first person in our family to hear those words. At the time, they still hadn't been able to locate my parents.

"You need to get here right away."

I walked back around the stadium and some good friends were there. It was devastating. Coach Sloan told my buddy Greg Flanagan, "Go with Nick to Tennessee."

We went to the airport on the team bus, then caught the next flight to Johnson City. I was very emotional, but I still didn't know how bad the situation was for Marc. I didn't know he was fighting for his life. I didn't know he was on a ventilator. I didn't even know the nature of the paralysis. Was it permanent? Was there hope that he could recover and walk again? I knew what the doctor had said, but I didn't understand the gravity of the situation.

I didn't have a cell phone. I didn't know how to get ahold of my parents. I had a credit card for emergencies. I booked two seats on a flight to Johnson City, Tennessee, to see my little brother.

Chapter 19

The Call: New Jersey

DAD: Every weekend Terry and I went to see whichever of our sons' teams was playing at home. It was either Durham to see Nicky play, or Charleston, South Carolina, to watch Marc's game. That day the boys had away games. That's what made the day with Richard so relaxing.

I met Richard Catenacci for the first time at a pizza joint in South Bend one night after preseason practice. We were tired of eating cafeteria food. There were six of us sitting around having a Coke, eating pizza. The bill came, and it was twelve dollars. The other guys were arguing over who had two Cokes and which one ate more pizza. Richard and I looked at one another, reached into our pockets, pulled out two dollars each and threw it onto the table and told the rest of them that we'd see them later.

Rich was 5-foot-5 and weighed maybe 135 pounds. He had a very good voice and he ended up being in the glee club. We became fast friends that night. He lived down the hall from me in the dorm. He was rooming with a guy who was disgusting; the guy smoked and hated his parents. He had a picture of his father on a bulletin board and he'd throw darts at it. Richard was afraid he'd wake up one night and find the guy trying to kill him. I wasn't enamored of my roommate either because he thought he was all-world. Turned out the guy never played a down at Notre Dame.

One day I told my roommate, "Look, this isn't working out. You are going to have to move." I arranged things so that he would move down into Rich's room and Rich would move in with me. We became very close friends and our relationship has lasted throughout our lives. We took every vacation together. When I started playing professional ball we'd go up to Vermont to ski. I couldn't ski, of course, because I didn't want to get hurt. Richard would come with Terry and me on a ski vacation. It would be the three of us in one room. Richard would be on one bed, and Terry and I would be in the other. He came with us on just about every vacation all over the world. He became Uncle Rich to the kids. He's a wonderful, generous man.

Every year at Notre Dame I'd get my game tickets before the season started. I sold them right away for $500. Back then, $500 was a lot of money. I took the money and I put in my toiletry bag. Periodically Richard would run out of money. He knew where I kept my money. He'd take a ten or a twenty, and put an IOU in its place. Then at the end of the month he'd put the money back in. He is just so dependable and trustworthy.

Terry and I were enjoying our time with Richard at his New Jersey farm when his brother, Peter, came back out onto the terrace where we were sipping our champagne. He told me I had a phone call.

"Nick, the chairman of the board of your company is on the phone and he has to talk to you."

I was president and chief operating officer of U.S. Tobacco, a Fortune 500 company. If I was out of the office, I always left a number where I could be reached. This was before cell phones and the internet, much less text messages or e-mail. I thought something had happened either in Washington, D.C., or at the state level with regard to the business.

I got on the phone and Lou Bantle said, "Look, Marc's been hurt. This doctor has been trying to reach you. Please call him right away."

I had no idea what had happened. I thought Marc might have hurt his knee or injured his shoulder. I knew he had a neck and shoulder problem because I had been on the phone with the Citadel trainer and the team doctor earlier in the week. Both of them assured me that Marc was fine. What the doctor said was, "We're going to take care of him."

I dialed the number Lou provided and reached the doctor. The first words out of his mouth were, "Your son dislocated his neck, and he'll be a quadriplegic for the rest of his life."

I literally went to my knees. It was such a devastating disclosure. And the stark delivery on top of it.

"Get here as quick as you can because your son is dying. *Your son is dying*. Get here as soon as you can."

My first thought was, "How do I tell his mother that her son is dying?"

Chapter 20

Into the Void

MOM: I think I had my second spiritual conversion very young. As a nurse, you are faced with the reality that some things are out of your hands. Most young kids don't think about death and dying at that age, but I was confronted with it every day when I was twenty-one.

My first surgery I held a leg while it was being amputated. That was my first scrub in the operating room. It was draped, but I was holding the leg as it was being cut off. I think faith is a gift. I find comfort in prayer.

I was still sitting out on the terrace admiring the view and drinking my champagne when Richard came out to get me. He took me into a room and there was Nick, sitting on the floor. He was a mess. Nick was crying and barely able to stand up.

As a nurse, I knew too much. I was better than Nick in the immediate crisis, but all I kept saying to myself is, "He's still alive. Where there's life, there is hope."

Chapter 21

The Call: Gainesville

GINA: I was working at Macy's in Gainesville talking to a co-worker about how accident-prone my family was.

My brothers were always in the hospital getting stitches. I had been kicked in the face by a horse. Marc and Nicky never wore shoes even when we played kick-the-can at night. One night, Nicky tore open his leg like a zipper from the ankle to the knee. Marc cut his head jumping on the bed. A car hit him when he was younger. It went on and on.

I was having this hour-long conversation laughing about all these incidents when I saw my roommate coming down the escalator in the store.

"Renee, what are you doing here?"

She's a very sensitive person, so it was hard for her to say the words.

"Gina, you've got to . . . Um, come upstairs and take a break for a minute. I've got to tell you about something."

Then, when we were alone: "Something happened to Marc. You have to call your parents."

I could tell by her voice that this wasn't just another clumsy moment in the Buoniconti household. My first thought was that Marc was dead. I found a pay phone and called my parents.

My mother said, "Oh my God, it's Marc. It's Marc."

"What?"

"He broke his neck."

They had called my apartment, where they reached Renee. I was in the midst of the conversation about all the injuries, stitches, and hospital visits when Marc broke his neck. By the time Renee found me, it was just thirty minutes after the injury. Marc was still on the field.

My mom didn't know if he would live. I remember saying, "He's going to live." It was a blur. This was my little baby brother. He was coming to Gainesville the next week to visit me.

We all got to Johnson City quickly. But it was grim, really grim. Marc didn't look bad. He looked like Marc. But, oh my God! I kept telling myself, "He's going to walk. This is temporary. He's going to walk."

He had a halo on. He was in traction. He was on a respirator. No one knew what to do. My dad was pacing. Nicky slept the entire night right next to Marc. It was just so emotional seeing my baby brothers side by side all night, and no one knowing what would happen.

Chapter 22

Breathless

I thought, "Don't panic. Don't freak out, man. You just broke your neck."

I couldn't breathe. It was that sensation of having the wind knocked out of you with no ability to get it back. It was actually due to the dislocation of my neck. I was fighting for every breath. No matter how hard I tried, I couldn't catch my breath. The first people to approach me were our team trainers. I couldn't communicate. I tried to speak but I didn't have enough breath to make a sound. I'll never forget the golf ball-sized eyes with which they gazed at me, full of uncertainty and bewilderment. It was their eyes combined with my lack of sensation that confirmed what I already knew. I began to feel myself going in and out of consciousness. Later on, they told me I turned blue on the field. How I didn't suffocate is a miracle.

The elevated neck roll and the straps connecting my shoulder pads to my helmet made me vulnerable. The contraption restricted my neck from extending backwards. Our necks are designed to withstand impact and many more pounds of pressure when they have an opportunity to extend backwards. Neck injuries are much more prevalent when the head and neck are forced to flex forward. Try rocking your head slowly backwards and you'll be fine. There's flexibility there, and range of motion. Then slowly move it forward. The range of motion is much more limited. The amount of pressure you're able to withstand diminishes with the head and neck restricted.

My neck dislocated forward. It was pushing against my larynx and throat. I was gasping for air. I knew I was hurt badly. There were no sounds. The once exuberant crowd went from roaring and cheering to looking on in complete silence. Not only was the sound gone. Everything moved in slow motion. I have no idea how they got my helmet off without killing me. They taped me to the spinal board. I lay on the field for thirty minutes before they loaded me into the ambulance. Once in the ambulance I tried mouthing to the paramedic, "I can't breathe." He tried using a nasal cannula—the small flexible tube placed under the nose with the two prongs that go inside the nostrils and deliver small amounts of oxygen. I remember looking at him, as if to communicate, "Are you kidding me? I don't think that's going to cut it." By the grace of God, I made it to the hospital, still alive.

The last thing I remember clearly was arriving at the hospital in Johnson City. As they were taking me out of the ambulance the first doctor said, "We've been expecting you."

The staff was coming toward me with a large hose covered in lubricant to intubate me for a respirator. I instinctively opened my mouth to receive the tube but I heard them say: "No, this goes in your nose." I couldn't believe it because it looked the size of a garden hose. They pushed it up my nose. I could feel pressure and tremendous discomfort, as it pried open my nasal passage. As the respirator tube went down my throat I started throwing up. Once the respirator was hooked up, the machine began breathing for me. I could feel sensation in my face and shoulders, but nowhere else.

In my periphery I could see two doctors reviewing the results of my X-rays and scans. They turned to me. The first thing they said was that I dislocated my neck and damaged my spinal cord.

"You are paralyzed. You may not be able to ever breathe on your own without the assistance of a respirator. And you'll never walk again."

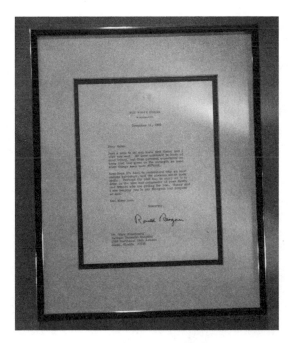

A December 1985 letter from then-President Ronald Reagan

An October 1986 letter from former President Richard Nixon

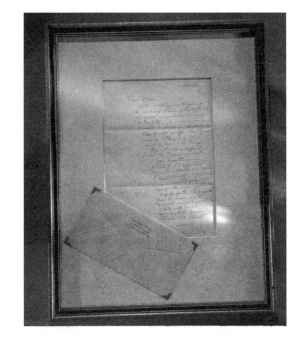

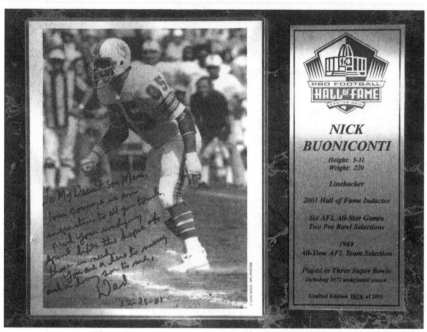

A Nick Buoniconti autographed photo, personalized to Marc

A December 2006
picture of Marc with
his mother Terry

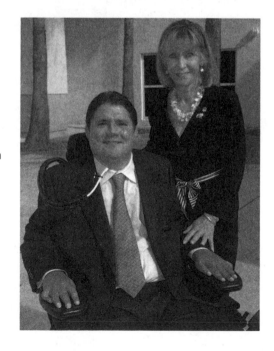

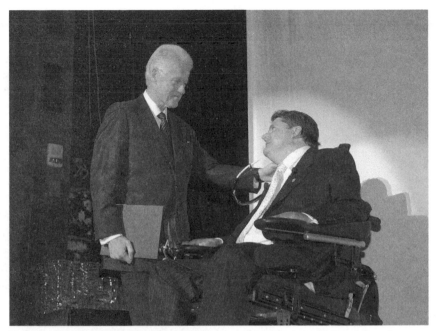

Former President Bill Clinton with Marc at the 25th Annual Great Sports Legends Dinner in September 2010

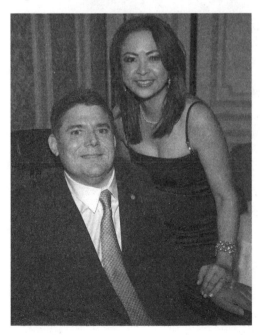

Marc with his fiancée Cynthia Vijitakula at the 30th Annual Great Sports Legends Dinner in October 2015

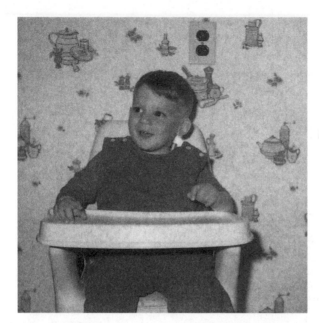

Marc as a child

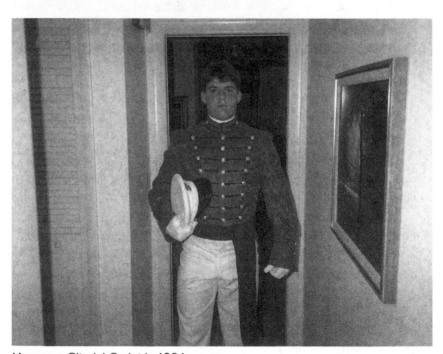

Marc as a Citadel Cadet in 1984

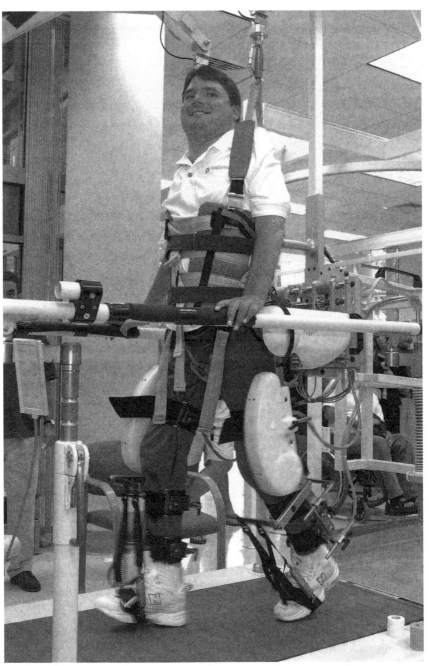

Marc on a robotic walking system at The Miami Project

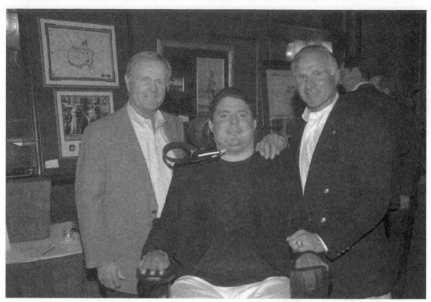

Golf legend Jack Nicklaus with Nick and Marc in 2004

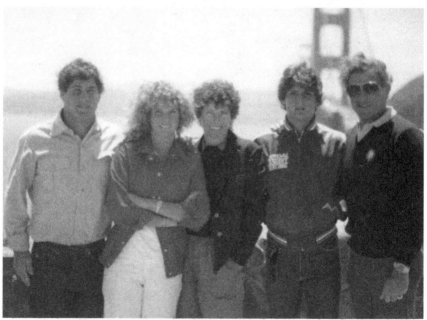

A Buoniconti family trip to San Francisco in 1982

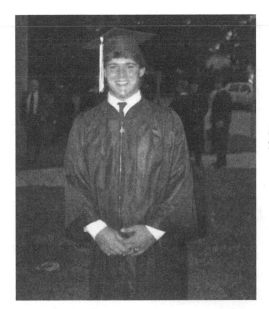

Marc as a Columbus High School graduate in 1984

Marc with Nick at The Citadel in 1984

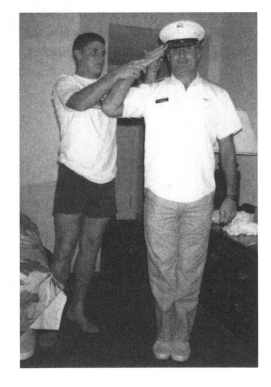

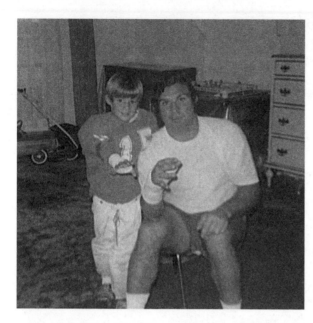

Marc comparing injuries with Nick in 1972

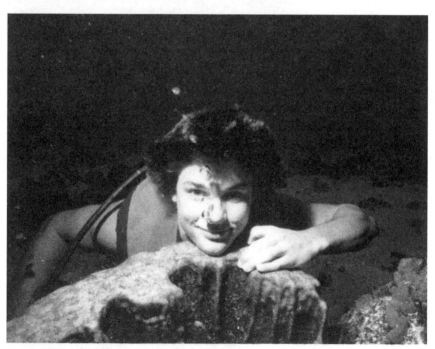

Marc SCUBA diving in Miami as a teenager

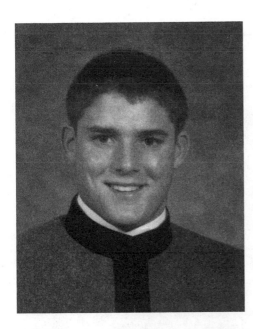

Marc as a Citadel Cadet
in 1984

Marc playing
football at The
Citadel in 1984

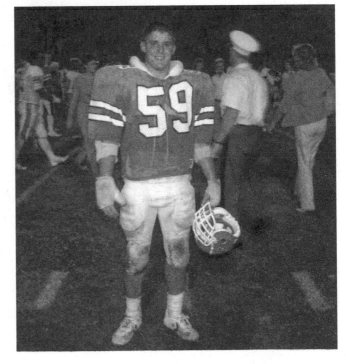

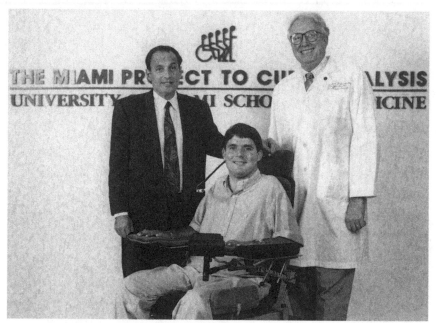

The Miami Project co-founder Dr. Barth Green with Marc and The Miami Project Scientific Director Dr. Richard Bunge in 1989

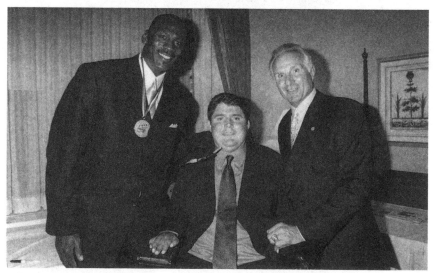

NBA legend Michael Jordan with Marc and Nick at the 2000 Great Sports Legends Dinner at New York City's Waldorf-Astoria Hotel

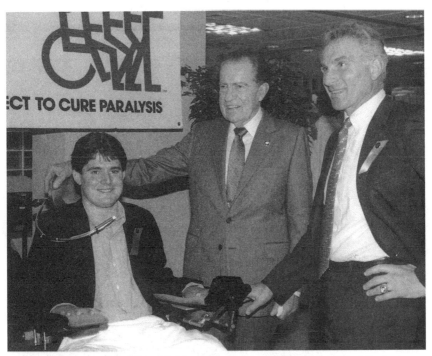

Marc with former President Richard Nixon and Nick at The Miami Project in the early 1990s

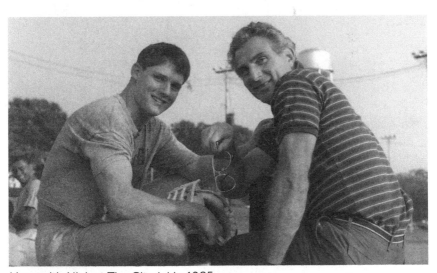

Marc with Nick at The Citadel in 1985

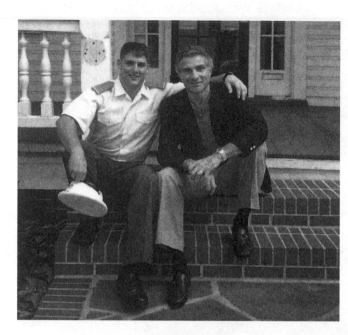

Marc with Nick
at The Citadel
in 1985, two
weeks before
he was injured

Nick with Marc at
The Citadel in 1984

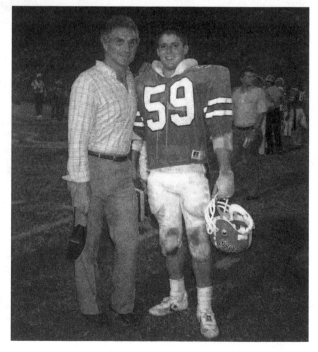

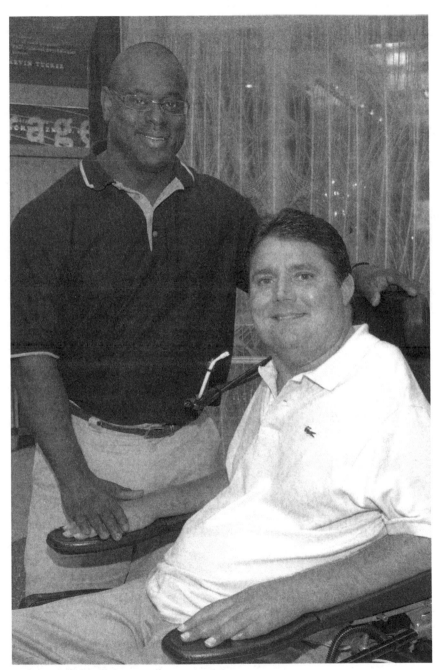

Herman Jacobs with Marc at The Miami Project in 2007

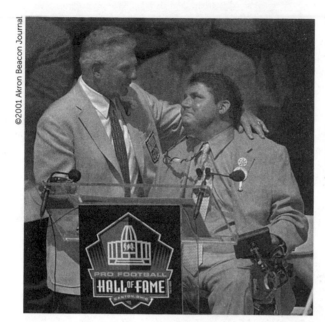

©2001 Akron Beacon Journal

Marc and Nick at the NFL Hall of Fame in Canton, Ohio in August 2001.

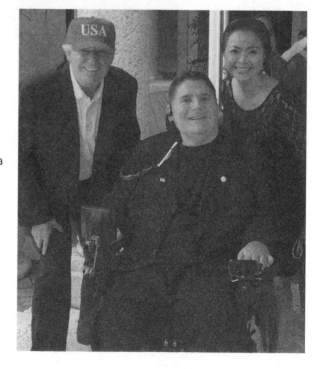

President Donald Trump with Marc and Cynthia Vijitakula at Mar-a-Lago in February 2017

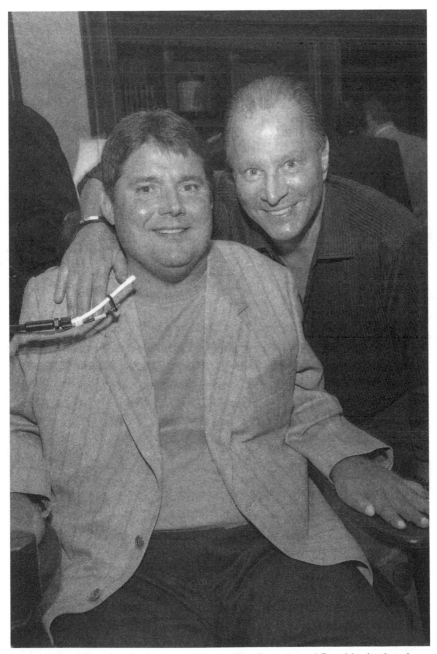

Marc with philanthropist Stewart Rahr at The Buoniconti Fund Invitational
Golf Tournament in April 2008

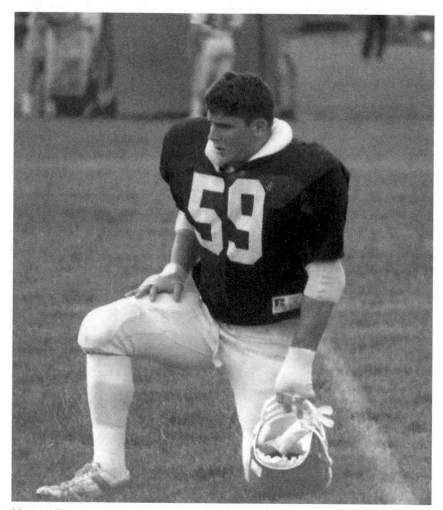

Marc at The Citadel in 1985

Part II

INTO THE DEEP

Chapter 23

No Way Out

NICK JR: I didn't get to Johnson City until around 8 p.m. I knew Marc was hurt badly, but I'm not sure what anyone could have said to prepare me emotionally for the scene. The more people I saw as I walked into the hospital, the worse I knew it was for Marc. Sometimes the unknown is scarier than reality because of how our imaginations twist pieces of disconnected information. Not this time.

When I walked into the room, it was awful beyond my imagination. Marc had tubes coming out of him everywhere. He was connected to a machine that was breathing for him. And he was unconscious. Emotionally I was blown away to a degree I had never experienced. I broke down crying along with my mom, my dad, and my sister. We all cried uncontrollably as Marc lay there in silence, unaware of all of us falling apart around him. He was on the edge between life and death, and none of us could do a thing to pull him back.

The people at the hospital were great. They just weren't equipped for someone hurt as badly as Marc.

Neither were we.

Chapter 24

The Hard Part of a Simple Game

I have barely any recollection of what transpired during the forty-eight hours following the injury. I was in and out of consciousness due to all the medication. I recall sporadically seeing each member of my family come into the room; I couldn't tell you who arrived first or what they said to me. It was all a haze. All I knew for sure was that my family was by my side that night. The rules for "visiting hours" didn't apply. My sister and brother spent the first night with me in the room. At that point, it wasn't clear at all whether I would make it through that night alive, much less beyond that.

From what I was told, my brother came into the room and nearly tore the place apart. Here was a guy who had worked so incredibly hard for everything in his life. He studied hard, smoothed out any physical deficiencies on the football field with tenacity and hard work to become a starting linebacker for Duke. Then he walked into a hospital room where his little brother was fighting for his life, and there was nothing he could do about it. No amount of hard work, not a single ounce of intellect was going to change what had already taken place. I would have felt much the same way, particularly at that time. I always believed, and still do to this day, that I can do anything. And I pretty much did right up until the moment I could no longer breathe on my own or move a muscle in my body. In the blink of an eye, any semblance of lingering resentment from our tumultuous past faded. Rather, what surfaced was the ever-present emotional connection of brotherly love.

I was told that my dad tried to pry off his Super Bowl ring. As he saw his youngest child struggling to survive, my dad felt betrayed. A game that had given our family so much, now was taking something away. A cooler head prevailed as my mom stepped in to head off any unnecessary rage. As devastating as the situation was, the fact that it happened on a football field wasn't lost on my father or brother. My dad's career began there and our lives grew out of what he did in the game. Football didn't define us, but it was a common bond with a language and a culture understood by our entire family.

The game of football provided my family with so much, including our greatest joys. And now—grabbing heaping handfuls of what it had given—our greatest sorrow.

I'm sure the situation would have been no less traumatic if it had been, say, a car accident. But the fact that it happened the way it did made the cut deeper. It would make the wound that much harder to heal.

Chapter 25

Help Me

DAD: Marc was literally dying when we reached Johnson City.

They had him hooked up to everything imaginable. He was heavily sedated. He also was dying right in front of us because his lungs were filling up with fluid.

I looked into his big brown eyes. Marc couldn't talk. All I saw in those eyes was Marc telling me, "Daddy, please help me."

For the first time in my life I couldn't help my son.

Chapter 26

The Promise

Another moment that seemed inconsequential amid the chaos would prove to have a profound impact on our lives and the lives of many others. It was a grand gesture, one that only a parent would make in the face of pain and desperation.

My father simply said, "Marc, I promise that I will do everything in my power to help you walk again."

Little did we know at the time that those words would become our mantra, and the life force of our yet-to-be-discovered future.

Chapter 27

What's Next?

GINA: Nicky was upset and very angry. The fact they couldn't do anything to help made the situation intolerable for him and my dad. It was terrible. Virtually every minute of the first twenty-four hours, my father and others were on the phone trying to find the best doctors for Marc.

The hospital was brand-new. It just wasn't a place for someone with Marc's injury, particularly in 1985. Eventually, it came down to New York, or Miami and Dr. Barth Green. At the time, Dr. Green was a young neurosurgeon.

My mother was amazing. She was like a Red Cross nurse on the battlefield, a woman in her element. She's the one who held everyone together in those first days and nights.

My dad was angry, very angry. He was like a caged animal. He needs to have control, and he couldn't control anything.

Chapter 28

I Need to Save My Son

DAD: We knew very quickly that to save Marc's life we had to move him.

The first person I called was the team doctor at Duke. I knew him, and I knew Duke had a great medical center. I talked to people at Yale, the National Institutes of Health. There were a lot of other people making phone calls for me as well. Remember, this is before the internet or cell phones.

Finally, the Duke doctor said, "One of the great trauma centers in the world is the University of Miami/Jackson Memorial Hospital. There's a great doctor there named Barth Green, who is probably one of the best spinal cord injury doctors in the world."

Chapter 29

Emotional Triage

MOM: I was pretty good in the immediate crisis. Marc was heavily drugged. There weren't any bruises or cuts. He looked the same. He looked like Marc.

When Nick and I were in high school, a young boy broke his neck playing football. He died within a year. I remember the kid being in a bed that continually moved him around to keep the fluids in his body in motion. The bed was called a Stryker frame. It's an incredible piece of equipment, but the hospital in Johnson City didn't have one.

Within twenty-four hours, the pulmonary specialist put everything on the line.

"He's already getting pneumonia," he told us. "If you don't move him, then he is going to die."

We looked all over the country, and we kept hearing about this Dr. Barth Green in Miami. We lived in the city, and we had no idea. I was going to go wherever Marc went. We decided Dr. Green was the right person and University of Miami /Jackson Memorial was the right place.

Normally they would stabilize a patient's neck, particularly one with Marc's level of injury, before moving him. The slightest bump or movement could kill him. But Dr. Green didn't want Marc stabilized, which was fine with me because the hospital in Johnson City didn't have that capability anyway.

Marc's neck was still dislocated when the medical team arrived from Miami. One of the doctors in Tennessee kept telling us Marc couldn't be moved in his condition. He said Marc would die before he ever made it to Miami unless his neck was stabilized. But we listened to Barth Green, whom we had never even met before.

An anesthesiologist arrived, along with another assistant. They put Marc into a contraption that allowed him to be moved and ultimately put onto a plane so he could be flown to Miami. The anesthesiologist put Marc to sleep to keep him as quiet as possible. Simply moving him was dangerous. Travel came with its own risks. But those risks were relative. We knew he wouldn't last long if we didn't get him to a major trauma center.

I flew with Marc on the medevac plane while Nick went with the other kids in a separate plane.

On this small plane, I held the IV for Marc all the way to Miami. I think I had been up for seventy-two hours by the time we arrived.

Chapter 30

Lost in Space

About the only clear memory I have of the first three days in Miami is when I arrived. I vaguely remember being moved from the airplane into the ambulance that transported me to the hospital. I knew what had happened. Time had no context. It wasn't clear to me how many days had passed or what day it was. Tubes connected me to a ventilator—a large machine with a mind-numbingly monotonous sound, without which I couldn't breathe. More than thirty years later the sound of that machine still has a particularly haunting effect on me. I can feel my anxiety level start to rise the minute I hear the whirl of a respirator, even though they're much smaller now, and less imposing than the one I had.

The first emergency surgery involved the removal of bone chips and the stabilization of my neck by fusing my fractured C-3 and C-4 vertebrae. Even though I was fully paralyzed, just the thought of undergoing surgery seemed to provide hope that my traumatic injury could somehow be reversed. This first surgery went well, but it didn't change my neurological status, which involved the obstruction of electrical impulse transmission through the damaged nerve cells in the injured section of my spinal cord. The dislocation of my neck caused severe inflammation and hemorrhaging of the spinal cord. The progression of the inflammation led to further damage, destroying nerve cells along the way. The initial trauma created a cascading effect from the release of toxins throughout the spinal cord which, when exposed to this hostile environment, undergoes apoptosis. That's a biochemical process of programmed cell death (PCD). My paralysis was caused by the combination of inflammation and damage to the nerve cells.

I was heavily medicated and the sensation was so disorienting that I didn't know for sure where the fog ended and reality began. It was like being lost in space. Days later, after the first major surgery to stabilize my neck, I clearly recall the sensation of moving through the air—at one point hanging upside down, and then rotating until the other side of the room was revealed. I was still unable to speak so I devised a rudimentary way of getting the attention of the medical staff by making clicking sounds with my tongue, like one makes when calling a horse. It was my only form of communication. Days later that clicking sound saved my life. A respiratory therapist turned off the ventilator alarm, which was the routine procedure when cleaning or replacing the tubing. The therapist forgot to turn the alarm back on. A little later the tube became disconnected and I began to suffocate. This got me clicking as loudly as I could, which drew the attention of a nurse who finally walked by my bed and noticed what had happened. She saved me.

As I floated I tried to deal with the strange sensation of flying and the dispiriting reality of what had happened. A nurse approached and I mouthed, "Where am I? What is going on? Why am I moving?"

The nurse told me I was in the neurological intensive care unit at the University of Miami/Jackson Memorial Hospital. He explained how long I had been there and reminded me of what had happened. I still didn't understand why I was moving. I didn't know whether I was hallucinating or, in fact, floating in the air. It turned out I was moving thanks to a special bed called a Rotorest. The bed is designed to move from side to side constantly to help mobilize secretions from my lungs and to improve the circulation of blood throughout my body.

Over time the monotony of it all pushed me to limits I didn't know existed. Initially, though, I remember being perpetually thirsty. I felt like I was literally dying of thirst. I couldn't drink anything at the time due to the respirator, which blocked my esophagus. All fluids came into me intravenously. The only way to alleviate the thirst was by moistening my lips with lemon-flavored swabs. Among the many strange and isolated memories of those early days was seeing an IV bag full of fluids on top of a dresser next to my bed. Every time the bed shifted me back to that side of the room, I'd see the bag again, and the thirstier I became. It was all a very surreal experience.

For a quadriplegic the complications accumulate in a non-linear fashion. A second surgery was initially delayed because a sore was discovered on my neck. I am susceptible to infection on all fronts, particularly with regard to my skin. When the sore cleared up and surgery was rescheduled, another problem was discovered. They found what was essentially a hole in the back of my head, which was due to rubbing back and forth against the bed.

These were the first, though certainly not the last, wounds I had to deal with. When I arrived in Miami, it took sixty pounds of traction to keep my neck aligned. The weight was attached to "tongs," which are actually ice-pick-like spikes that had been drilled into my skull. I had that procedure done twice, once in Tennessee, then again in Miami. One of the tongs actually popped out of my head at one point and the pain was excruciating.

The ICU of any hospital is a nasty place to be. It's particularly so in the Neuro ICU of a major metropolitan, trauma center. There were beeps and whistles going off constantly at all hours of the day and night. Those sounds blended in with sirens and the dull whirl of various machines. The entire place was brightly lit with no walls, only curtains sectioning off one patient from another. The sound of those curtains being drawn was just another noise amid the cacophony.

Around the clock nurses, interns, and doctors came into the room to poke and prod patients, most of whom were on the verge of death. Sleep was virtually impossible. The action was nonstop. New patients arrived, the deceased departed, and the specter of emergency was ever present. I was rotating side to side so I saw everything.

One night, they wheeled in a guy who had been stabbed in the eye with an ice pick. Doctors couldn't remove the ice pick because they were afraid he would die instantly. He ended up dying anyway, one of many who passed away around me in those first few weeks. To those around me, he became known as "Ice Pick Eddie," though I never really knew the guy's name.

There was so much death around me that I had to find a way to deal with its constant reminder. I didn't feel like I was ready to die. I didn't want to die, but death seemed to be lurking all the same. I'd see the nurses come in and slip another body into a bag just a bed or two away. I'd wonder if I would be next. I was consumed with trying to understand what was happening with my body, and whether the shadow of death would envelop me as well.

* * *

MOM: It was all so overwhelming in the beginning.

I didn't know what to pray for.

Do I pray for Marc to live, or do I pray for him to die?

Here was this kid who had been running around his whole life. How was he going to survive being forced to be still? What was his quality of life going to be?

A psychologist came to the room one day. The rest of the family didn't see the benefit of talking to someone, but I spoke to her a couple times. She said, "You won't believe the quality of life Marc can have."

"No," I told her, "I won't believe it."

That was my little boy lying in a hospital bed, respirator-dependent and clinging to life. I prayed for strength to accept whatever came next.

Chapter 31

Game Over

DAD: Marc was playing a violent game. A lot of things can happen in that game. One of them is paralysis.

If an individual dives into the surf without realizing the waves are going out and he hits his head and becomes paralyzed, that's totally unexpected. It's not necessarily expected you will get hurt playing football, though there's certainly a much greater likelihood of that happening compared to surfing.

We all know there is risk associated with playing the game. Becoming injured and paralyzed is the greatest fear that football players have. That's why guys who have neck injuries often retire rather than extend the risk.

I don't know how I avoided serious injury when I played. Maybe quickness had something to do with it, or the fact I played with good people in front of me. There's no one answer why someone like Jim Otto ends up having a leg amputated and all I had were two hip operations. Was it good fortune, luck? Who knows?

In my opinion, Marc's injury was a combination of incompetence and poor judgment by the trainer, doctor, and coaching staff. You put all three of those conditions together in a violent game and the odds of injury change dramatically. Marc never should have been playing in that game.

His neck was definitely injured. They had to create a contraption to keep his head in place. They knew he was hurt.

The point is that there was a greater likelihood that Marc would be paralyzed in that game than any other player playing that day at any level. If you put a kid in that position, something bad is going to happen.

I knew Terry couldn't live with the thought of another son taking that risk ever again. I went to Nicky, and I said, "I know you only have four games left. This has been so important to you, but I don't know how I can tell your mother that you are going to keep playing. It could happen. You could end up with the same injury as Marc, and we'd have two sons paralyzed. I really don't know if she could ever survive that. But it's up to you. You have to do what you feel is the right thing for you. It's your life. You have put a lot of effort into playing. It's gotten you to where you are at Duke."

I thought Nicky made one of the most unselfish and courageous decisions I have ever seen. He had to return to Duke and tell his coach that he would no longer be able to play because of what happened to his brother. That was an incredibly unselfish act.

* * *

By the end of the first week the morphine was wearing thin. The world began to slowly come into focus. The tears seemed to come in waves, often without warning. Everything about the situation was fragile. Everyone was emotional all the time, particularly my mom. Through the disorientating haze of drugs and a flying bed, I could see she was having a hard time coming to grips with the entire situation.

My mother had been a nurse at a young age, so she knew a lot about the critical nature of my condition. I recall looking into her eyes as she sat next to my bed. I noted how red and swollen they looked from all the crying. I became aware of how physically and mentally worn down she was from the stress of the previous six or seven days. If she slept, it was only out of pure exhaustion. The adrenalin was running low, and reality was pushing harder and harder into each day. By the end of that first week, we all knew that at some point soon my father would have to go back to work. My sister would return to the University of Florida. Nicky would head back to Duke and the football team.

I'm sure my mom recognized that at some point crisis would devolve back into everyday life, however different it might be in form and texture. She knew that it would be the two of us, together once again.

That last bit of reality was too much for her though. I recognized as much even amid the fog of my own emerging reality. The idea of another son going back to the scene of the crime, so to speak, was not something my mother could process. It was the first time, though not the last, in those early weeks and months, that we switched roles. I don't remember exactly what my mom said, but she made it clear to me that she didn't want Nicky to play another minute of football. I knew then that she wanted me to tell him.

My father made it through football relatively unscathed, thanks to his intelligence and tenacity. Nicky hadn't been nearly as lucky, though it never showed on the field. He had surgeries on both shoulders and played with a blown out right knee, along with countless dings, bruises, and body numbing "stingers."

I knew my mother was having a hard time. I also knew she couldn't bring herself to make the request. My mother told Nicky, "Your brother wants to tell you something."

I called Nicky over to the bed. As the bed moved back and forth, I mouthed:

"We don't want you to play."

Had it been up to me, I never would have asked that of my brother. But my mother was an emotional wreck, and I was afraid for her. You had to appreciate the atmosphere. Everyone was crying all the time. I was crying too.

To this day I regret asking Nicky to stop playing. I've never told him that, but it's true. If he had been injured like me, would I have stopped playing? I don't think so. Still, I regret asking that of him because I knew how much we all loved the game. I'm not sure what it would have taken for me at that time to unilaterally decide to not play. I felt like I let Nicky down by asking him to walk away from football, especially since he had only four games left in his senior season.

I knew my mother did not want him to play. What was I going to tell her? "No, let him play?" I was emotional myself. I was trying to console her because I knew I had to. I don't remember whether Nicky agreed at that moment, but I do recall that my mother, in tears, barely able to get out the words, said: "Thank you, Marc. Thank you."

Nicky went back to Duke, and he never played another down. At the end of that 1985 season the team gave him a plaque as the "Most Inspirational Player." He dedicated it to me, his little brother. I have it on the wall in my office to this day, a little plaque that says, "For Marc."

I'm not sure Nicky would have had a chance to play at the next level, but we'll never know. He was a hard-nosed player who played above his physical stature. He wasn't the strongest or fastest guy, but he was smart and very tough mentally, a lot like my father in those respects. He was all-out, all the time, and he never flinched on the football field. I know one thing: Nicky was as tough as anyone he ever played against.

It happened to be a unique time in professional football. There were more options for players coming out of college because the United States Football League (USFL) was around, in addition to the Canadian Football League and the NFL. We'll never know what the future might have held for Nicky. Regardless of what could have been, it was my injury and my request that sealed his football future.

At some point early on the trainer from The Citadel football team, Andy Clausen, came to see me at the hospital. He was crying, along with the rest of us in those days. I could see that he felt terrible. Likely, seeing me, in his mind, confirmed his worst fears about being responsible for the injury. I looked up at him and mouthed, "I don't blame you. I guess the contraption didn't work."

I knew he felt responsible. He did make a mistake, but he didn't do anything purposely to hurt me. He's actually a really nice guy whom I considered a friend. I was injured a lot so I spent a lot of time under his care. At the same time, I was struggling to survive. I wasn't focused on who was to blame for what happened to me, or really much of anything other than staying alive.

In late November or early December, my dad came to my room and told me that I shouldn't have been on the field that day based on the history of my injury. He told me then that we would have to sue The Citadel. He laid it all out and explained what would happen. He prepared me for what was ahead. I understood, but I had no idea then of the repercussions of that decision. I also didn't have the capacity to worry about it. For the most part I really just didn't have an idea what it all meant.

As the reality of my situation settled in, I told my family that everything would be OK. I didn't know that, but I didn't want them to keep coming into that room day after day staring at me and crying. I needed them to get on with their lives. I would have to do the same if I was going to survive.

Eventually my father had to return to work. UST was very gracious in allowing him to commute between Connecticut and Miami. You have to understand my dad. He would have been much more of a pain being around the hospital all day. He would have been looking for something to do, or to rant and rave about something that wasn't being done. The stress wouldn't have been good for any of us. It was better to have him return to work and allow life to get back to the new normal.

★ ★ ★

NICK JR: It wasn't easy having a conversation with Marc. His bed moved side to side, and he couldn't speak. I knew what he was trying to convey to me. I saw his lips move as he mouthed the words, but I didn't need to see them. I could see it in his eyes.

At the time, it wasn't a hard decision for me given the context of our lives. All I thought about from the moment I woke up until the moment I went to sleep was Marc. We were all there just about every minute of every day.

There was another paralyzed patient in the bed next to Marc. No one ever came to see the kid, so I made a point of visiting him every day. Then one day, he was gone. He had died.

The gravity of Marc's situation was sinking in slowly, but the tears, particularly my mom's, never stopped flowing. I could see the pain and the fear. Her eyes were so red, and she was worn down by the trauma. It was an easy decision. I imagined her sitting next to Marc's hospital bed on a Saturday afternoon for four hours wondering about her other son on a football field somewhere and waiting for the call to confirm that I had made it through the game. I couldn't put her through that.

If I had been a great player anticipating making it to the professional level, I might have thought twice about playing. But I was a 5-foot-9, 200-pound, relatively slow inside linebacker. When you are that age you think you can hang the moon and nothing can stop you, but I have always been a realist. I knew how good I was. I knew that at my size there wasn't a future beyond Duke.

My dad gave me more of a choice. He said, "In the end it's up to you whether you want to go back and finish the season."

The fact I wasn't playing anymore didn't hit me until I stood on the sideline for a couple games. It was that feeling of knowing there is nothing I can do to help my team. I knew they understood, but it still felt like I was letting all of them down. Standing there in street clothes was tough if for no other reason than what it represented. Marc and I started playing football when we were seven years old. The game was part of the fabric of our family. Now it was part of our identity in a way that no one could have envisioned.

The week I returned, Duke was playing Georgia Tech in Durham, North Carolina. Bill Curry, the coach at Georgia Tech, was coming off a tough stretch of games in a high-pressure job. But he walked all the way across the field and made a point of seeking me out.

"I just want you to know that our entire team, all of our coaches, everybody at Georgia Tech is praying for your brother."

That was a classy move by Coach Curry.

* * *

Nicky and Gina went back to school, my dad went back to work, and my mom and I were left together. This is the same woman that I had butted heads with on a daily basis for most of my life. Now I was completely reliant on her. To one degree or another, she was reliant on me too. All the bad grades, late nights, skirting around the edges of legal trouble, all of that disappeared into the past almost as if it had never happened.

Tragedy has a way of focusing every aspect of your being on what's truly important—family, health and, for a parent, the life and well-being of a child. Everything else falls away. We were all now in uncharted waters.

Chapter 32

The Inestimable Dr. Green

DAD: I really didn't meet Dr. Barth Green until a day and a half after we got to Miami because Barth was caring for Marc. He was in surgery almost from the moment we arrived at the hospital. I'm not sure whether it was six or eight hours, but with all of Marc's pulmonary issues and other complications, I didn't get a chance to sit down with Barth for at least the first thirty-six hours.

That's when Barth casually mentioned that there really wasn't enough going on in the world of spinal cord injury research. The only thing I knew about Barth, which helped endear him to me, was the fact that he saved my son's life. Everything was happening so fast. It wasn't clear what needed to be done, or what could be done in terms of finding a cure and funding research. The first two weeks were a blur because we were with Marc at the hospital eighteen to twenty hours a day.

At that time there were a couple of young, local kids who had been injured and paralyzed. One was the son of a doctor. The family was devastated. Barth had to go in and console them. He said, "I'm so tired of going into a room and telling families their child will be paralyzed and confined to a wheelchair for the rest of his life. I'm just sick of it. If we could raise a million dollars, I bet we could help put this thing behind us."

We pulled together the first fundraising event less than two months after Marc was injured. American Express came on board. We asked the Dolphins if we could have people going through the stadium with hat in hand to ask for contributions. Dick Anderson, my Hall of Fame former teammate, led the event. Whatever contributions we received, U.S. Tobacco agreed to match. We raised $300,000. That's how we started.

We all knew a million dollars wasn't going to do much, but it was a start. I had no idea where this would go from those first conversations with Barth. We were dependent on certain individuals to make our dream credible. There was nothing much going on in the world in terms of scientific research. We were starting from a blank piece of paper. We were trying to build an organization that until that point didn't exist anywhere. Every aspect was a question mark. Who are the scientists? Where are they now? There was no one in the world doing research at the level necessary to make a credible impact. There were pockets of work going on, but it wasn't very concentrated. No one believed a cure could be found.

The consensus was that it wasn't possible. So why would you spend time, money, and effort on something that can't be done? Imagine taking a telephone cable and cutting it in half. Suddenly you have hundreds of loose wires. Now you have to try to match them all up with the other side to put that cable back together in a way that energy flows through it just as it did before it was severed. That's what we were facing with spinal cord injury, only exponentially more complex. How could we ever begin to dream that we could fix that telephone cable?

Marc needed some reason to hope because at the time there wasn't one. I think all of us were looking for one as well.

Then one day, Marc told me that *Inside the NFL*, the show I did on HBO, was his favorite television show. He wanted me to go back to work so he could watch it. I couldn't bring myself to leave him until he told me to go back.

It was reassuring. Marc felt comfortable that he was going to live.

* * *

When I first met Dr. Barth Green, I was so heavily medicated that it was a blur. Over the next several weeks, as the fog began to lift, he checked on me daily. Dr. Green was a positive energy force in an otherwise

dismal environment. He had a presence about him that was conta-
gious. The one thing I knew for sure was that the guy loved sweets.
My room was filled with baskets of candies, chocolate, and all sorts
of goodies, and when Barth came to visit, he raided the stash like an
addict. But he was determined in his pursuit to provide the best care
for me, and his other patients. You could see right away that this was
the kind of guy you would want to have as your doctor. He always had
a smile.

One day, I heard him and my father mumbling about a vision that
Dr. Green always had. Imagine, each and every day having to break
horrible news to so many families. Barth was disappointed in the
field of neuroscience and the lack of progress in spinal cord injury
research. Up to that point, paralysis due to spinal cord injury was a life
sentence, with no chance of recovery. Most people stayed at home or
in nursing homes. In many cases hope was reduced to hoping to die.

Barth explained to my father that if we could raise enough money
to bring together some of the best scientists in the world, then we could
create a multidisciplinary approach to spinal cord injury research. We
could find more effective treatments and ultimately, a cure for paralysis. Barth thought of the moonshot project and the Manhattan Project
and how, through a collective effort of desire, funding, and teamwork,
anything was possible. Hell, if man can walk on the moon and har-
ness the power of the atom, then surely, we can cure paralysis. Thus,
The Miami Project to Cure Paralysis was born.

I needed a reason to look toward the future. However, there was
one giant obstacle: getting off the respirator. The only hope to regain
any sense of freedom and independence was to breathe on my own
again.

Of course, that was easier said than done.

Chapter 33

Walking into the Future

MOM: I don't think Nick could deal with the day to day. Mothers are a little different than fathers. We take things however they come, which is not to say Nick felt any differently about Marc after the injury. It's just that mothers see things from a different angle.

Here was Nick, a father with two boys who grew up to be accomplished linebackers just like their famous dad. Nick had that deep pride in his sons just like his father and grandfather had in him when he was growing up. He was proud of what his boys were able to do on and off the football field.

I've always thought that when Marc got hurt there was someplace inside where Nick blamed himself.

Chapter 34

Another Pain in the Neck

The second surgery took place in November. Barth was concerned that there were additional bone chips producing unnecessary pressure against my spine. It could have been related to my diaphragm's lack of function. This time Dr. Green went in through the front of my neck. My injury is near the top of my spine. A dye was injected above the injury. Dye lights up the X-ray if there is a blockage. That's all fine, but when you have an injury like mine, the area above the paralysis is hypersensitive. I can feel everything above my shoulders, so I had to be given morphine before the procedure. Not even morphine blunted the pain, though.

First, a sheath or guidance catheter was inserted into the side of my neck. I felt everything from the initial puncture all the way into my spinal canal. They didn't come close to getting where they needed to be to inject the dye. The catheter needle was already deep into my neck when they realized it wasn't long enough. They must have used a nine-inch needle. They didn't take into account the fact my neck was a thick, muscular nineteen inches at the time. So they took out the shorter needle, got a longer catheter, and then started the entire process over again. I have experienced a lot of pain along the way, but that was the worst pain I have ever endured. The procedure went on for an hour. I cried through every minute of it. It seemed like it would never end and the intensity of the pain never lessened. Pain is hard to describe. That was beyond anything I could imagine. I have no idea how I was able to hold on without passing out.

My life did pass before me, but not in the ways you might expect. In between the surgeries and the constant attempts to keep me stabilized, I tried to come to grips with the reality of my situation. I thought about everything in those first six weeks. It was intimidating and I was afraid. I had no idea what was happening to me, or what was lurking just around the corner. I remember the only other time I felt intimidated by anything. I was one of the youngest freshmen at Columbus, only thirteen when the school year began, so you can imagine how big the seniors seemed to me. They were huge. Football practice started a couple weeks before classes. We weren't even wearing pads and the older guys looked like grown men. One of the varsity running backs was sweating so hard that he had foam coming off his face and chin strap. I thought, "Holy Christ!"

To that point I had never been intimidated by anything or anyone other than my brother. The coaches asked each of us where we wanted to play, offense or defense. I told them I wanted to play tailback on offense and middle linebacker on defense. That was a mistake. There were a lot of guys in the linebacker group. Most of them were big guys. I ended up splitting time between tailback and linebacker. Instead of gaining the knowledge of both of those positions, I was learning half of each. As a result, I wasn't proficient in either one. Also, I was not getting sufficient repetitions in either group.

The coaches didn't give a shit about me. I was just a little freshman. I probably weighed 140 pounds. It was a strange feeling. For the first time in my life, I felt out of place on a football field. I didn't spend enough time with either position to gain the trust and confidence of the respective coaches. I was frustrated and really upset. What made it worse is that a friend with whom I played Pop Warner football was starting ahead of me. He was a little bigger, but in all fairness, I didn't think he was better than I. The year before, in Pop Warner, he actually played the slot running back, which is not a primary position for carrying the football. Now I was the one standing on the sidelines. The entire situation was disorienting.

I told my dad, "I can't handle sitting on the bench watching someone who isn't better, playing ahead of me on the field." My dad encouraged me to keep working hard. He also said that I should consider going back to the Pop Warner League because I had another year of eligibility. I felt dejected. I was losing my enthusiasm for football. Eventually I went directly to the JV head coach. "You know, Coach, last year when we won the championship that guy played behind me. Now I'm here standing on the sidelines." If he had a response, I don't remember hearing it. I pushed on, "Coach, I know you have no reason to believe me but come out to a Pop Warner game and watch me play." He never did.

I decided to do what few had ever done at Columbus. I went home after high school football practice, got on my bike and rode to Pop Warner practice. I decided to use that last year of eligibility. I wore my Columbus football gear to Pop Warner practices and games. The only thing I changed on game days was my helmet and uniform. In the first Pop Warner game, I was just killing guys. But it wasn't the same. I felt like I had graduated from that level, and it was hard to stay motivated because of what was happening at Columbus. It showed during a game against the South Miami Gray Ghosts. They had a good running back. On one play, the quarterback pitched to the running back, and the guy was hauling ass around the corner. I was playing middle linebacker. I could have gotten him, but I totally loafed. I gave up on the play.

My dad never missed a high school game, and he rarely missed a Pop Warner game. He had never said a word to me before a game, one way or another. If I wanted to talk about something that happened in the game, then he would listen. He never critiqued my play or made a point of telling me what I did right or wrong. This time was different.

When he saw me give up on the play, he came out of the stands, all the way out to the sideline, grabbed me by the facemask, and said, "You're playing like a fucking pussy. All these kids are looking up to you, relying on you to be their leader. You made a commitment to them. And you're playing like a fucking pussy. I'm not going to let you do it to them. You either play the game the right way, or I'm going to drag you off this fucking field!"

According to my teammates, what happened next was one of the most memorable moments for anyone at that game. The opposing team had just scored a touchdown. I went back out onto the field as the kick returner, with the full fury of having been reamed out by my father. The ball came to me. I locked my arms and ran as fast and hard as I could. Three guys came up to hit me. Bodies went flying, complete with equipment, shoes, arm pads, helmets. One of my friends described the scene as a bowling ball scattering ten pins in a bowling alley. Put it this way, they had to stop the game and carry three guys off the field. I was the only one who got up on my own, but I was buzzed the rest of the game. I definitely had a concussion. I'm sure after my dad saw that, he knew the message got through. He never had to say anything like that to me again. The experience knocked some sense into me.

My dad never cared whether we won or lost. It was all about effort. He didn't tell us to "go out there and win." But he did tell us never to quit. The expectations he had for us were the same he had of himself. Give a hundred percent effort, at all times. That's all he asked.

That was a life principle that helped sustain me in the hospital. I knew that the quality of my life depended on me getting off the ventilator. The life expectancy for someone with my injury on a ventilator is no more than ten years, which is exactly how long Christopher Reeve lived.

Chapter 35

The Sights and Smells of Death

NICK JR: The ICU was a strange and depressing place. It was loud all the time. There were at least a half dozen people in various forms of trauma, a number of them paralyzed just like Marc. The place had its own smell to go along with the odd assortment of noises.

At least once an hour, and sometimes two or more times an hour, a nurse would pull back the curtain. It was time to clear the mucus from Marc's lungs, or what they called "suctioning." He had to be taken off the respirator while a long tube was inserted into the hole at the front of his neck.

Marc gasped for air. He couldn't get an ounce of oxygen. When they finished, he was hooked back up to the respirator. It took a few minutes before the terror in his eyes subsided. It was one of dozens of issues Marc had to deal with, and this one seemed to happen constantly.

* * *

MOM: We have always said that Marc is the only one in the family who could have survived this.

Gina and I have said we aren't strong enough to deal with that level of injury. We'd probably be dead. Nick couldn't do it, and my son Nicky probably couldn't do it either. Marc is the only one. He could do anything when he set his mind to it. He just didn't set his mind to the things I wanted him to when he was younger.

But that same kid was still there. He couldn't breathe. He couldn't even talk, but he still had that sparkle in his eyes.

I remember Dr. Green saying one day, even as Marc lay in bed unable to move and hooked up to all those machines:

"I know he can't move, but I keep feeling to make sure I have my wallet."

Chapter 36

Thin Air

Before Gina and Nicky returned to school after Thanksgiving, I told my brother that by the time he returned for the Christmas holidays I'd be off the respirator. I didn't even come close. I was out of the woods relative to the injury, but the hardest part of the first year was still ahead of me. I was stable enough to know I wasn't going to die due to the injury, though there were all kinds of complications created by my condition. Any of them could kill me at any time, so I was still struggling.

Dr. Green made it clear that I had to get off the ventilator. He wasn't going to allow me to deviate from that goal. Inflammation discovered during the second surgery effectively confirmed what the doctors feared. I wasn't going to get off the machine anytime soon, if ever at all. Dr. Green never wavered, though. He knew it was my only chance. If he had any doubts about my ability to breathe again it never showed. He was relentless and completely unyielding no matter what I said or how much I complained.

The monotony of it all was getting to me. I could see that my mom was still having a difficult time coming to grips with the situation. Between Thanksgiving and Christmas, we both started sinking under the weight of reality. I was going through the first psychological

166

stages, made famous by Elisabeth Kübler-Ross, of someone undergoing a traumatic experience—anger, denial, bargaining, and depression. I certainly never believed in the final stage—acceptance. I didn't want to accept the realities associated with my injury. I felt this would constitute a kind of defeat since it would make my condition irreversible. I felt that once I accepted the situation, then I had already given up. I wasn't even sure I would ever be able to break free of the respirator. One way to check breathing ability is by measuring what is called "tidal volume," which is the volume of air available in your lungs. I had zero.

In an attempt to train my body to breathe again, Dr. Green set the respirator to a certain number of breaths per minute. To wean me off the machine that number was slowly and methodically reduced. What was really being reduced was the available air. Instead of taking ten or twelve breaths per minute, like a normal person, the machine was set to provide me only nine or ten breaths. Then it dropped down to eight, seven, and so on. The object was to make the body so hungry for air that it would respond by trying to breathe on its own.

It sounds good in theory. In practice, it is no different than being slowly and yet constantly pushed to the edge of suffocation. Frankly, it freaked me out. I was wide-awake watching the clock, counting down the seconds between breaths. I figured out the setting on the respirator. I recounted quickly in my head. Was it eight breaths per minute, or seven? How long did I have to hold my breath before I could receive another one? This went on twenty-four hours a day.

By the time I got down to six or seven breaths a minute, it was equivalent to torture.

Chapter 37

I Couldn't Move, Either

MOM: One at a time they left. Gina went back to the University of Florida. Nicky went back to Duke, and Nick returned to work. It was time, I knew. But that's when the heaviness of it all hit me. I was exhausted. I was scared for Marc more than anything. I cried an awful lot.

The reality of Marc's situation really came into focus when everyone left again after Thanksgiving. I realized that this was going to be Marc's life. The intensity of the stress, the lack of sleep, everything caught up to me. I was exhausted in every way, even spiritually, you could say.

Then, I just couldn't get out of bed.

It took my dad coming over to the house one day. I couldn't move. I was laid out in my bed crying. He came into the bedroom. This is all he said: "Have faith."

Thirty-two years later I still get emotional thinking about his words. He hit the nail on the head. You either have faith, or you don't have faith. It's either there, or it's not. Faith is a gift. My dad was quiet in terms of religion. He'd go to church, but he didn't talk about it very much.

But it was my dad who got me out of bed.

Chapter 38

An Injured Warrior on the Battlefield

DAD: Within six weeks of Marc's injury, The Citadel stopped communicating with us, except through lawyers. That's why we all ended up in court.

To me this was an easy situation to resolve. All the school had to do was to stay committed to Marc. That's why I had a very tough time even years later when Marc reconciled with The Citadel.

I'm an Italian kid from the south end of Springfield, Massachusetts. I knew the right thing to do. It was obvious. They chose not to do it. Instead, they left a wounded soldier to fend for himself.

To Marc's credit, he did. I never told Marc what sport to play. I never told him what school to attend. There are a lot of things I never told Marc. But I did tell him that it was his decision if he wanted to reconcile with The Citadel, not mine. It took nearly two decades and the great effort of his friends to make it happen.

You know, their motto is they never leave one of their own on the battlefield. I've always said they left one of their soldiers on the battlefield when they turned their back on Marc.

Chapter 39

The Angel Rode a Harley

When I moved into a regular hospital room, which was just down the hall from the ICU, I got my own private nurses. James "Jim" Escoto was my daytime nurse and, for me, an angel disguised as a drill sergeant. I saw Jim every morning. That's when all the therapy took place—the chest pounding to clear my lungs, the stretching of my limbs, occasional bathing, and so on.

Jim was a former Airborne Ranger. He served in the Army but also had been a mercenary—a "freedom fighter"—in Nicaragua during the Sandinista-Contra war in the early '80s. He was a womanizer and a real man's man. Jim was an outdoorsman and a scuba diver. He rode a Harley Davidson wearing a Nazi army helmet. He was a tough guy, and he didn't put up with any of my shit.

Jim got me up every morning. He literally dragged me out of bed. There is no doubt he came into my life when I most needed him. He was military tough and psychologically even tougher. I was comfortable with all of it because I had seen it before at The Citadel, though at times I hated him. He wasn't very big, maybe 5-foot-7, with dark hair and a mustache. But he was physically fit with a wild streak. Jim followed his own code. I respected that. More than once, though, I threatened to fire him because he never gave in to my complaining.

He wouldn't let me quit no matter how much I bitched. Everything he did was in my best interest even if I didn't recognize it at the time. Still, one day I told my mom, "Tell Jim not to come back." She said, "You tell him." And that was that.

I also had a physical therapist, Paul Kleponis. Every day he and Jim transferred me from the bed to a chair. I passed out every time. "Take a deep breath. Pretend you're going down for a lobster," Jim would say. "See you in a minute." They would disconnect the ventilator and I'd pass out. The next thing I knew I was in the chair. That happened every day for months.

It was like God sent this man down to be my drill sergeant. He was no different than Dan Bridges and the other upperclassmen at The Citadel. It was my worst nightmare all over again. Deep down, Jim had a great heart. He knew what I needed to survive. If I didn't get off that respirator, it wasn't going to be due to a lack of effort on his part. Still, the confinement and complete lack of independence started to wear on me mentally.

I was attached to the respirator. The machine was large. There were hoses coming across my body. The sounds were unnatural. There was a constant feeling of something tugging on my throat; it was the pressure from the respirator pulling on the tracheotomy tube. Then there was the constant chest therapy and the suctioning of my lungs. All of it started to wear me down. The suctioning happened fifteen to twenty times a day around the clock. A nurse would remove the respirator and slide a tube into my trachea or through the hole in my neck down into my lungs. It was like a vacuum that sucked out the mucus and saliva. I had to hold my breath until the process was complete and the tube was reconnected. Meanwhile, the bed never stopped rolling side to side. Condensation would regularly build up in the hose and then drip into the trachea, which made me feel like I was drowning. The worst part was that every once in a while the hose to the respirator would just pop off. Then I had no air at all. I would click as loudly as I could to get the attention of anyone. When that happened, I was terrified. Without the respirator I knew it was only a matter of minutes until I was dead.

I did have the perfect training for all this. I grew up in my mom's Polish training camp with all the discipline she demanded. I learned the meaning of never quitting from my brother and my dad. Everyone in our family is driven, so I was exposed to that philosophy as a matter of course from an early age. Then I went to The Citadel with all the training, running, and discipline. Psychologically, mentally, and physically, I was as prepared as anyone could be. Still, fighting that machine was harder than anything I could have imagined.

I had promised my brother that I would be off the respirator by the time he came back for Christmas break. By the time Christmas was over I wasn't even close. When everyone left after the holidays, I was drifting. I couldn't see any light at the end of the tunnel. On the contrary, it seemed to me that I was only getting worse. I had tubes in my nose, down my throat, and I was strapped down like Frankenstein on a moving bed. I could feel myself going down. I couldn't eat. I couldn't speak. I was losing weight and I was depressed. The denial was gone and reality arrived in waves of despair.

I thought Dr. Green was being unreasonable because he didn't realize the torturous nature of what he was doing to me. My mom was trying to encourage me to get off the respirator. I didn't think anyone understood what I was experiencing. I really didn't think they appreciated, nor could they understand, what was happening to me. Imagine being suffocated for the majority of minutes every hour and no one acknowledging that it is happening. I mouthed the same message all the time: "I can't breathe. You're killing me."

I woke up every morning with tubes coming out of me. The beeps, the sounds, and smells of the hospital were constants. The bed was a version of water torture all by itself. People were touching me all the time—poking and prodding me for some reason or another. There wasn't a thing I could do about any of it. Depending upon the day, they came in to announce that the intensity of the torture was about to be increased. "OK, time to lower your respirator."

At some point I had been reduced to seven breaths per minute. Then it was lowered to six breaths, which meant one breath every ten seconds. I was sinking. I had no idea how far down the bottom was.

* * *

MOM: I still didn't know whether to pray for him to die or to live. He was still on the respirator. Then he got that "decapodous ulcer" (pressure sore) on the back of his head. The only thing he could move was his head, so the back of his head rubbed against the bed so much that it created an ulcer.

A young nurse who took care of Marc was crying, "We didn't even think about the back of his head." She was so upset.

On top of everything else, Marc now had what amounted to a large hole in the back of his head. The doctors had to debride the area, which means they had to go into the ulcer and cut it all out. There had to be pain associated with the ulcerated area, but Marc never said a word. That just shows you how much was going on with his body at the time. There were so many serious issues that it was overwhelming even to that poor young nurse.

My nursing background was the biggest help and to some degree the biggest hindrance. I had taken a refresher course a couple years earlier, so I was current with the technology and nomenclature. That knowledge provided a level of security particularly after we arrived in Miami. I remember Nick wouldn't leave Marc's room because he was afraid somebody would miss something that Marc needed. I knew enough to know that Marc was safe at Jackson.

Then again, a little knowledge was dangerous too. In some ways, I knew too much about what was happening to him.

There are just so many issues facing a person in Marc's condition. I came into his room one day, and he was delirious. It turned out that his bones were losing so much calcium that it was poisoning his body. Astronauts have problems with calcium release because of weightlessness. It's truly a case of if you don't use your bones, then they slowly lose some of their integrity. So much calcium was being released into Marc's system that it sent him into delirium. I thought he might be having a stroke, or worse.

Nothing was easy for Marc. Arteries contain oxygen, and they reside deep in our arms and legs beneath veins and skin. It was critical to know how much oxygen Marc was retaining in his system. But the process of finding out was so awful. I sat there one day and watched them puncture

Marc's arm in search of an artery. It was so invasive. I thought, "Thank God he can't feel a thing."

Marc was constantly catheterized, so bladder problems became an ongoing concern. His blood pressure would shoot up or plummet. We knew that if he survived the first year, then his body would adjust. But the poor kid was constantly in crisis of one form or another.

Amid all that he battled the ventilator.

Chapter 40

Survival Training

I always felt as though my back was up against the wall. I had challenges, a lot of challenges growing up. I never had enough breathing room because I was always under stress and strain to conform.

I effectively learned how to swim with sharks in the middle of the ocean. I did it my entire life. I was used to living on the edge. I knew how to survive. Even at The Citadel, where the stress of school was compounded by the relentless intensity of my day-to-day existence, particularly as a freshman, I never lost sight of who I was. I persevered. I found a way through. It wasn't easy. It wasn't always the most efficient route.

Nothing I had experienced compared to the journey I started early in 1986, about three months after the injury. I started shutting down. Mentally, I crawled even deeper into myself. It's dark in there, man. We all have that place, but it's at a depth few of us want to dive down into. It was cold, dark, and entirely unlike life at the surface. No one goes there out of simple curiosity. In my case, at least, fear of the known, combined with fear of the unknown, produced a kind of energy that pulled me inward. As it was happening, I could feel my mind and body wasting away.

I saw the looks on my parents' faces when they stood beside my bed. I could hear the fear, if not the horror in my mother's voice as she begged me to eat. I had to retreat so that I could find the strength to face whatever came next. I knew I would have to do it by myself and on my own terms. I had to do it without the ability to do anything physically for myself; lacking the capacity to execute even the most fundamental assertive act—I couldn't breathe. There was little evidence to suggest that would ever change.

At the same time, I couldn't accept a life tethered to a machine. I had to confront the question of my existence. Did I want to live? Both figuratively and literally, I went into lockdown inside my hospital room. I was trying to find a reason to live, to carry on a fight while demons seemed to be multiplying and rising up against me. I was down to four or five breaths a minute. I became so deeply consumed by the process of trying to breathe that I was exhausted physically, mentally, and spiritually. Every moment of every day was the same to the point I couldn't see beyond the seconds ticking off the clock. Ten more seconds until another breath. Five seconds. Then, gasping, a shot of air would flow into my body. Then fifteen more seconds before I could get another one. I was experiencing what felt like the most inhumane form of torture, a slow death.

I couldn't see beyond the intensity of a battle within a war between the ventilator and me. The exhaustion was unlike anything I had experienced in the outside world. It enveloped every aspect of my being. I didn't want to be touched. I didn't want to be fed. I didn't want my face washed. I refused everything I could. I knew a patient had rights. I had the right to refuse care. For the most part that's what I did; maybe because that's all I could do. I couldn't handle any more distractions. Could I find a reason to keep fighting the fight? I really didn't know.

The fact that I wasn't progressing added to the gravitational pull on my soul. It sucked me deeper and deeper inside. I reached a point where there was nothing left to consider but the question of my mortality. Of course, that question had been there since the moment of the injury. For a long time, it hadn't necessarily been mine to answer. Doctors were in charge. For them, death is an outcome, not a choice.

Eventually, living or dying became the only question left. Honestly, it could have gone either way.

They were ready to insert what is called an "NG tube" into my nose to feed me. I had no appetite. I was being worn down. Every hour seemed to consume, almost literally, another pound of flesh. At one point I was down to 126 pounds, exactly one hundred less than when I walked onto the field in Johnson City, four months earlier. I could feel my body deteriorating, slowly at first, then with momentum. I listened and watched as my mother pleaded with me.

"Please Marc, please, you have to eat. You have to get your strength back."

She could see what I intuitively knew was happening. As bad as it was for me, it had to be awful for a mother to watch her child wither away right in front of her eyes. There was nothing she could do. I wasn't sure there was anything I could do either. Over time, I wasn't even sure I *wanted* to do anything. I never got to the point where I was ready to give up. It was more a matter of being unable to see any reason to keep fighting. No matter how hard I tried to breathe, nothing seemed to matter. The darkness continued to engulf me.

The realization that everything was beyond my ability to change began to set in. A sense of doom was like a constant darkening that overwhelmed any potential light. Hope was being extinguished. I began to realize that if there continued to be no progress, life would be taken from me.

I came to understand that choice itself was slipping away from me. I was trying. It just got to a point that defeat seemed inevitable.

* * *

DAD: Seeing Marc physically deteriorate was traumatic. I'd be gone a week, come back, and he'd lost even more weight. Watching him wither away in front of me was tough. There was really almost no reason for him to live until they started weaning him off the respirator. That was such a major ordeal, more psychological than physical.

I don't think I ever pushed Barth for anything other than getting Marc off the respirator. Barth was adamant about everyone around Marc, includ-ing the nurses, having a positive attitude. Everyone who had anything to do with Marc was instructed to be positive. I knew Barth was doing his part. But, Marc had to do his part too. Ultimately, he did.

Marc started to become more normal as he got closer to getting off the respirator. Until that point he had been rather abnormal. He was still going through all the emotions. The only time that I saw anger was when they lowered his breaths. When that happened, Marc really rose up.

It was easy for us to support lowering the breaths per minute. We didn't have any problem breathing. Marc was suffering. I remember when he got down to six breaths per minute. Marc was really struggling.

Chapter 41

No Direction Home

There was never any discussion, as far as I knew, about an alternative to getting off the respirator. If I was going to die, whether I liked it or not, they were going to make sure I died trying. No one, certainly not Dr. Green or my nurse Jim, was going to allow me to go quietly into that good night. In their minds defeat literally meant death. It didn't matter to them if it cost me another hundred pounds. It wasn't as if they were looking the other way, pretending there was progress when there wasn't. There were no delusions. They were resolute and committed. At that point, my choice was either to keep fighting, or submit to self-induced suffocation. In other words, I had to refuse to breathe. It could have gone either way. Either way wasn't going to be pleasant. The option of living on the machine was never offered. I came to know it never would be.

I had a very subtle sensation of improvement. It happened in what was perhaps the darkest series of weeks. Nurses came into my room to suction me. They placed the tidal volume meter on my trachea. I looked down at the gauge. I saw it move. I had always tried to breathe on my own in between the breaths provided me by the respirator. For the first time, though, I was able to get the needle to move. The nurses didn't even notice. So I gestured for them to put the meter back on and tried to breathe again. Sure enough, the needle flickered.

It showed about 50 cc of air, which is like a small syringe-full. I couldn't believe it. In an instant I could see the slightest glimmer of light. I mouthed: "Did you see it? Did you see it? That's air! That's air coming out. On my own!"

The nurse very calmly replied, "Yes, that's air."

It was a defining moment, and it came at a time when I needed it most. I needed a sign that I could improve. When I saw that I was forcing air out of my lungs on my own, it was the first sign that I had a chance against the machine. That's when I started coming back to the surface. However slightly, the fact that I moved the needle inspired me to breathe as hard as I could. For the first time since I started my descent, I saw the possibility of life. That night, when my mother came into the room, I mouthed the words, "Look, look. I can get a little bit of air out."

It wasn't enough air for me to survive. But it was as if everyone understood the sign. I'm not sure anyone around me ever lost hope, but my recovery had been re-energized. Every day from that moment forward I tried to extend the time I was off the respirator. In retrospect, the swelling related to the initial injury no doubt had started to sub-side, which is likely why I was now getting some air. I was fighting so hard to breathe that even the slightest effort started to produce results. I had been breathing by pulling myself up with my shoulders and my neck, which created negative pressure to assist the diaphragm in expanding the lungs. My accessory muscles were suppressed by the inflammation, which in part was why it was so difficult to breathe. At the moment of my injury, I couldn't move anything, including my shoulders. Inflammation is an immediate and overwhelming response to catastrophic injury. It's also why people often die.

I drew on every experience in my life. I needed every bit of it to survive. I relied on the drive that is part of my family, the toughness of my mom and my brother, the power of my own personality. I relied on the chip on my shoulder that helped me through every challenge. I never thought I would encounter a test beyond the experience of my freshman year at The Citadel. That paled in comparison to beating the respirator. The school trains you to overcome unwinnable situations. I was taught how to react and adapt to situations that a normal person wouldn't be able to navigate. Ironically, my greatest physical feat was accomplished at a time when I couldn't move.

I went from the edge of death unable to move, unable to draw a sustaining breath, to finding the courage and drive to make the choice to move forward. My body could have gone in the other direction at any moment. I knew that if I could get off the ventilator it would change my life. All it took was the slightest movement of a needle. I'm not sure I would have survived if I missed that sign. It provided me hope at a time when there was no reason to have any.

That month taught me more about myself than anything I had ever experienced. For most of my life I relied on family, friends, and coaches. The battle with the respirator was an intensely personal fight that took place in the deepest recesses of my being. I never had a spiritual awakening. Nothing close to a moment when I saw the white light or felt the hand of God. But I do know it was a mental and physical battle that exceeded anything that had come before in my life. It was about redemption. It was about life. Maybe I needed to descend into the deep to appreciate the possibility that I could have a life, even though there was a great chance that I'd never be able to move.

From the moment that I saw the needle flicker I started to improve exponentially compared to where I had been. My volumes went from 50 cc, to 100 cc, to 200 cc and so on, until after a few weeks my volumes reached 500 cc. That's when the discussion began to remove the trach-tube from my stoma—the hole in my neck—to allow my tracheotomy site to heal. It was another indication of my progress. I wasn't quite ready for that, though. I had to understand that even though I hated the trach and the ventilator they provided me with a sense of security.

Eventually, I began to breathe on my own all day long, which required strenuous effort. At night I went back on the respirator so I could rest. I was terrified of falling asleep without the respirator, then suffocating. I told my mom my concerns, and she assured me that she would stay by my side. She wouldn't let anything happen to me. One afternoon I happened to fall asleep. When I woke up I realized an hour had passed. I had survived on my own.

Seven months after my injury I was finally off the ventilator. I still had the trach, but I began experiencing the first real sense of freedom.

Chapter 42

A Band of Buddies

NICK JR: My buddies and I would call Marc almost every day when I returned to school in the spring. I knew he was struggling and it was painful to watch him fight to breathe. We were seniors, so it was a party every day at Duke. No more football. No more training. Most of us barely had any classes.

None of my friends ever lost sight of what was going on with Marc. We celebrated every five-minute increase in the time he was off the respirator. If I called the hospital and my mom told me Marc was up to fifteen minutes, then everyone would crowd into my room. We'd have a party and call him. It went on like that all through the spring until he was off the ventilator for good.

My dad is tough, and my mom is even tougher. I don't know if any of us are any tougher than Marc, though.

That's why his nurse, Jim, was so good for him. He talked right back at Marc. They would fight and argue. Jim wasn't going to let Marc talk him out of what had to be done. In so many ways he was the perfect guy. We all felt exactly the same way. Barth Green was a hard-ass too. He knew more than anybody what it meant if Marc didn't get off the ventilator. He refused to allow that to happen.

Then there were Marc's friends. They were as much a part of his recovery as anybody else. It was like a band of war buddies being around them. Most of them were kind of still hanging around Miami. A couple went to college, but that ragtag group had a remarkable bond. Every time I showed up at the hospital one of them was there with Marc. None of them blinked when it came to his injury.

For those guys, nothing changed. Marc couldn't move, and he was confined to a hospital bed, then a wheelchair. For those guys, Marc might as well have had a paper cut. Their relationships, their bonds never weakened. He needed all of that.

* * *

It's often said the fortunate can count one or two real friends in a lifetime. I have been blessed with countless good friends, many of whom I consider family in the deepest meaning of the word. I have never stopped being actively engaged with life and people across all walks. Those experiences introduce me to people who play significant roles in my life.

That's how life is. Sometimes you choose your friends. Sometimes circumstances choose them for you. Yet, true friendships are defined by shared values that are often taken for granted because they have been there from the beginning.

Sometimes it takes a tragedy or an extreme challenge to elicit the essence of those characteristics—companionship, compassion, honor, loyalty, and a deep familial-like love.

As soon as I arrived in Miami, certain visitors were allowed to see me. It's as if my closest friends that very day made a lifetime commitment to care for me, to make sure that I would be OK no matter what challenges I might face in the future. There was never a moment that my friends weren't by my side, literally and figuratively. Despite the whirlwind around me, they provided a sense of normalcy that carries through to this day. My friends have played the metaphorical role of my backbone through years of continuous and consistent support. Friends visited me, if not daily, then weekly. Each brought their unique personality.

One instance always brings a chuckle. In late December 1985, just a couple months after my injury, two of my friends, Willy Pierson and Scott "Dodie" DeNight, came to visit. I still had tubes coming out of every orifice. Willy walked up to my bedside, and with all sincerity said, "So, Markie, how was your Christmas?"

There I was practically dead and my friend drops the line of the year. I looked at Dodie. He could see what I was expressing: "How do you think my fucking Christmas went?" It actually made me crack a smile and provided me a sense of normalcy that was nonexistent at the time.

A few months later, I ventured outside the hospital room. I sat in a courtyard and enjoyed the fresh air and sun. George Abaunza was one of my friends who never stopped coming by the hospital. He would even skip visiting his girlfriend, who worked at the University of Miami a couple of buildings away. He spent time with me instead, which infuriated her. George fed me my first Big Mac. He also brought me Nestlé $100,000 candy bars. We loved them and George brought one every time he visited. He became friends with my nurse Jim too. He helped Jim get me out of bed and into a wheelchair. Then he would push me around the hospital.

My trachea hole was pretty much closed by May 1986 because I was breathing relatively normally. One day while relaxing in the hospital courtyard with Jim, George arrived for a visit.

"Dude, my brother gave me some kryptonite." Pot? I didn't hesitate. "Jim? I'm going to take a little walk with George."

Jim didn't hesitate either. He knew he could trust George, who wheeled me across the street. We loaded into the parking garage elevator and rode up to the top floor. I had accomplished so much. I had beaten the respirator, overcome numerous close calls with death, and in my mind, it was time to celebrate. Even after everything I had been through, I was still me. So we lit up a joint.

I tried taking a drag, but couldn't inhale because of the trachea hole. I mouthed to George, "Put your finger over the hole." So he covered the hole in my neck, I inhaled, then he let go and a cloud of smoke floated out of my neck. I was laughing and gagging at the same time. George freaked out for a second until I gave him a nod and a smile to signal that I was okay. Now, I don't want you to think that George was a bad influence. The moment wasn't about smoking pot. It was about recapturing my sense of self.

We were good friends during high school, but in the years following my injury we developed a brotherly friendship to the point where my mom still refers to him as her "other son." I spoke often to George about my deepest concerns following my injury—mortality, religion, God, fate, destiny—the kinds of things I ruminate about daily now. George was studying philosophy, which made him a dependable yet critical sounding board. He went on to earn a doctorate in philosophy from Florida State University.

Smoking pot on the hospital roof with George was my coming-out party. I had formally returned to the world of the living. My friends heard that story and responded in one voice: "He's back! You're still Markie! We don't care if you're in a chair. We love you."

I was getting more pressure from Dr. Green and the staff to remove the trach. As I mentioned, having the ventilator was like a security blanket. I hated that machine, but I knew it kept me alive too. I was scared to take the leap and rely on my lungs full-time. If I didn't remove the trach, then I wouldn't be able to transfer to the Rehab Center. One morning all the docs came into my room and said, "Today's the day." What most concerned me was the potential inability to clear my lungs of secretions if necessary. I wouldn't be able to be suctioned without the trach access. The lack of a strong diaphragm meant my cough reflex was extremely compromised. The doctors assured me that by using a technique called "quad-coughing," I'd be able to clear my lungs. The technique involves someone placing a hand just below my sternum. In sync with my effort to cough, they push in and upward to increase the strength of my cough reflex.

Removing the trach was one of the most significant decisions I would ever have to make due to the tremendous impact it would have on my future. I figured Dr. Green had been right about everything else. He saved my life while putting my neck back together. He enabled me to breathe on my own again by facilitating what he knew was a necessary form of torture.

With some trepidation I relented. Five minutes later it was out. I had graduated to the next step in my recovery. It was one step beyond the nightmare I had been caught in for seven months.

In an instant I was finally awake.

Chapter 43

Everything Is Looking Up

MOM: Marc became a new person when he moved from the hospital to rehabilitation. He was still in the hospital, but he was off the ventilator.

One day I was standing beside his bed. All of a sudden I noticed something. I couldn't believe it.

"Marc, it works!"

"Mom, what are you talking about?"

"Look, you have an erection!"

I don't think it ever occurred to any of us that it was possible.

* * *

Moving to the Jackson Rehabilitation Center was a joyous occasion. At the time it was a twenty-four-bed facility located about two hundred yards from the main hospital. It represented a giant leap toward life.

Rehab consisted of occupational and physical therapy. There were various techniques including the use of a Swedish arm sling designed to improve my range of motion and strength. I also "stood" with the help of a tilt-table, which is a stretcher with a base on the bottom. I was strapped in and tilted upward in a standing position. The object was to help with circulation and thus improve my bone density. There were all kinds of classes on sexuality and emotional issues, all of them designed to prepare me for the next step, which was to leave the hospital for good.

I learned, and my mother happened to point out, that quads get erections. Needless to say, that was a revelation in form and substance. I wasn't exactly a saint in the hospital. After all, I needed some motivation. I had a few girlfriends visit. They willingly pulled their shirts up, or took off their clothes for my benefit. During my time in rehab probably a half-dozen girls were more than accommodating to brighten my spirits. They certainly provided a lot of incentive, that's for sure.

Movement of any kind depends on the level of the injury: the higher the injury, the less mobility. The first vertebra is located right below the head. All the nerves that come from the diaphragm meet in the neck, which means there is the possibility of breathing, albeit in a limited capacity. An injury at C3 (Cervical) means the person cannot lift his or her arms. They can move their head and shoulders, nothing else. As the injury site moves down the spine movement generally increases. Injury to C4 or C5 affects movement of arms and biceps, but not in the fingers or triceps. At that level, there is no hand dexterity. At C5 and C6 there is near full movement except normal dexterity in the fingers. At C6 or C7, depending on precisely where the injury is, the person might have use of hands and upper extremities.

An injury at T1 (Thoracic) means you are paralyzed from the chest down. The designation goes down to T12 in your lower back, then to L3 (Lumbar). That's why you'll notice certain paraplegics—especially those injured way down on their back—have legs that are completely flaccid, with no muscle tone. That's because the nerves going down their back, called the "horse's tail" because they branch out, have been damaged.

People like me, with an injury higher up the spine, which in every way is more catastrophic, means no arm movement. But we can still achieve an erection. Apparently, my arms aren't *that* important. Actually, that's not entirely true. I wish more than anything I could move them.

In any case, I started to realize there was a life to be lived. It might not be the life I wanted, or the life I thought I'd have, but it was better than the one I had on the ventilator, and certainly better than no life at all.

I left the hospital for the first time on September 29, 1986, my twentieth birthday. My dad and his friends pulled together the first major fundraiser for The Miami Project, the first Great Sports Legends Dinner at the Waldorf Astoria in New York City. After nearly a year in hospital beds, I spent my first night on the outside sleeping in a bed at the Essex House in New York City.

* * *

DAD: My upbringing informed everything I have done in my life. I saw a father get up at 5:30 every morning, seven days a week. Sometimes it was five in the morning and he wouldn't come home until at least six at night. He'd be dog-tired, exhausted. He was working to do what? He was working to put food on the table for his family. It wasn't about buying a new car or saving to buy a new house. There were no vacations. We never even went out to dinner. Growing up I can remember going to two, maybe three restaurants until I went to college.

My grandfather was the same way. He and my father used to go to work together. It was a work ethic. I never had to think about working hard. That's just what you do. To me it was a matter of doing what needed to be done.

I couldn't leave Marc out there on an island by himself. That's basically where he was. He was in uncharted territory. He was paralyzed. We weren't paralyzed. Marc couldn't move his arms or legs. It looked like a real dead-end street for him. There was no research and there wasn't much hope. It was rough.

When we started The Miami Project it represented hope. Not that there was much more than hope. We didn't have any answers. We didn't even have a game plan. But we knew what we wanted to do. So we made sure that when we named The Miami Project we clearly stated its mission—The Miami Project to Cure Paralysis. It wasn't to build a better wheelchair. It wasn't to provide comfort to the sick. That wasn't it. We were clear as to what we wanted to do.

The effect brought friends together. It was a tremendous amount of work by a lot of people. It really kicked off with the first of what became the annual Great Sports Legends Dinner in New York. It took place eleven months after Marc's injury. And Marc was there. He was alive. And there was hope.

Chapter 44

An Angel Gets His Wings

I became very close friends with my nurse, Jim. He was a huge part of why I actually had a life. We would hang out, have a beer, and talk about life. The best drill sergeant is tough because he's trying to make you strong enough to survive down the road. That's what Jim was to me. He helped save my life.

Towards the end of rehab, as I was getting ready to go home, Jim came with me to New York for that first dinner. He loved the whole scene, and we had a great time. When we returned, Jim began planning a coming home party for me. Here's the kind of guy Jim was. He was re-tiling the floors in his house, by himself, so that I'd be able to move through the party without a problem.

Jim would often talk about a particular neighbor and how they always argued. There were disputes ranging from the noise of Jim's Harley, to the fact that Jim would allow kids to pass through the easement between their properties to fish, to a hand grenade incident. Apparently, Jim threw a grenade into the lake behind his house one night, and it blew out all the windows in his neighbor's house. Even though Jim took care of the damage, the feud only intensified over time.

When we returned from New York, I went back to the rehab center. One night, I went to a reggae concert with some friends and another nurse. The nurse received a phone call during the concert. Suddenly, she started crying. It was that unmistakable crying that accompanies news of a death.

"Did someone die?"

"Yes," she said, "someone close to me."

Dr. Green's staff had told her not to say anything to me. I went back to the hospital that night, and early the next morning Dr. Green came into my room. He told me Jim had been killed. I was devastated. I could only imagine what happened. Jim was probably up at 6 o'clock in the morning cutting tile with a wet saw and his neighbor went nuts. Although no one knows what actually ignited the fuse, apparently the neighbor walked over to Jim's house with a handgun and started shooting at him. Even after he shot Jim three or four times, Jim was still trying to get away. He was still fighting for his life when he tripped and fell. The guy came over and, after having emptied his gun, picked up a large rock and repeatedly slammed it into Jim's head, killing him.

It was an extremely sad moment wedged into a time when sadness had only just begun to fade. It wasn't just me, though. Everyone who knew Jim loved the guy. It was terrible. At his funeral there was an open casket. Jim wore a headband with The Miami Project logo on it. That was it. He was gone and a week later I was heading home, without my friend.

One thing about life is that it always leaves you asking: Why do things happen the way they do? Jim was like an angel who dropped into my life. Then, when his good deed was done, God called him back home. Jim prepared me for my new life, and then he was gone. If it wasn't for Jim, I might never have gotten off the respirator. He was exactly the kind of man, the kind of person, I needed during this most challenging time in my life. There are certain individuals, teachers, coaches, or parents, who have a profound impact on our lives. He was one of those people. Jim had the military culture, and he was also a little off-center, just like me.

Jim's death was a jarring experience. I was reminded that I had been given an opportunity to live. And living was the task at hand.

The old Marc spirit slowly returned. As far as I was concerned, I had been grounded for a long while. My love of life and fun emerged once again and, against all odds, even stronger than it had been before the injury. I came back from the brink. I crawled right up to death's door, and then decided to find my way back toward the light. I was reborn. Not in the Christian "born again" sense but in terms of life itself. I came back from the edge. Now I was all about celebrating life, albeit all the wiser.

That's one reason people in wheelchairs, especially quadriplegics like me, are often the happiest people you'll ever meet. I faced three or four life-threatening episodes in the first year. There have been nearly a dozen in the years since. I learned how important it is to live for the day. I can't waste a single one because I never know how many I have available. We all know this. Yet we so easily forget.

Throughout that year in the hospital, and even in the depths of my battle with the machine, my mentality never changed. I always knew that I could do whatever I wanted to do. Now I had to do it differently, that's all. I have to live *this* day, *every* day, as it comes.

My friends never allowed the injury to change how they felt about me or how they expected me to approach life. Their spirit helped carry me out of that hospital room, through rehab, and into my new reality. They never let me miss a beat. There was never any discussion about what I could or could not do. It was full speed ahead, business as usual.

But it wouldn't have happened for me the way it did without Jim. I miss him because of what he meant to my life. Everyone misses Jim because of the kind of person he was to the world. He was an angel who came into my life for a moment in time when I needed him most and nothing less would have made such a difference. He helped me navigate a catastrophic event and the menacing machine that came with it. Jim talked me through the depths of my anguish. When I came out the other side, there he was, waiting for me.

Then he was gone. But apparently, that was enough for both of us. One way or another Jim trained me in mind and spirit. He was an authentic warrior in every sense of those words.

The only thing I missed about leaving the hospital and going home for good was that my friend wasn't coming with me. It's hard to reconcile the idea of his death. After a year of fighting, suffering, and ultimately prevailing, I was the one going home. I'll never forget Jim. Neither will anyone who had the pleasure and honor of knowing him.

* * *

MOM: When Marc made it into rehabilitation, I knew that at some point he would be coming home. At first I was terrified. As difficult as it had been for all of us, Marc far more than anyone else, of course, I always knew every piece of equipment he might need was nearby. There were specialists of every kind within minutes of Marc's room.

One day I approached Dr. Green.

"You know, Barth, I *am* a nurse. I can handle this. I can take care of Marc. We'll be fine."

"No, you are not going to be a nurse to Marc," Barth said. "It's very important inside a family that those roles are not confused. Marc has insurance. He needs registered nurses. I know you are his mother, but you cannot become his nurse too." I was always hovering, even to this day. But it was very helpful to hear those words from Barth.

I knew the house wasn't perfectly suited for someone in Marc's condition. For a while, the poor kid had to take showers outside because his wheelchair wouldn't fit into any of the bathroom showers. The same outdoor shower head we used to clean off the kids from the dirt, grime, salty canal water, and everything else, was now the same one he had to use to keep his body clean enough to stave off infection and all manner of problems that come with a person bound to a wheelchair.

We managed, but it was scary. Then one day it all changed! The tension of it all was suddenly released. I heard all three of them arguing. Gina and Nicky had graduated. In the summer of 1986 they moved back home so we could all be together. When I heard the three of them arguing about God knows what, I thought, "That's great! Everything is back to normal."

Of course, it wasn't that simple. When Marc first came home, he became very sick with a urinary tract infection. He is, of course, prone to those kinds of problems. He ended up right back in the hospital.

It was an adjustment for everyone, to say the least, a transition into the next phase, not only for Marc, but for Nick, me, and Marc's siblings. That's not to say this wasn't one of the most frightening times for me. With my nursing background, I knew too much about what I didn't know.

I recognized how fragile Marc was even when everything appeared to be fine. But we managed.

We found a way forward as a family. I guess in some ways we all followed Marc into a new life.

Part III

THE RISING

Chapter 45

Getting Schooled—With Girls!

Leaving rehab and returning home was like returning from war. Everything once so familiar looked a little different. It was all the same but somehow new again. Figuratively, at least, I had dodged a lot of bullets and spent a year crawling through land mines. I was thrown into a war zone and somehow, I came out the other side. Even Jim's death provided a parting lesson. It was as if I needed one last reminder that life is precarious and nothing is guaranteed.

I was different. The entire experience changed me physically. There was no escaping that reality. But I was home. It was time to celebrate. That might seem like a strange emotional response when you can't even scratch an itch. It's counterintuitive. More than ever, I could choose to live for the day or choose to be miserable. The important thing, as we so often fail to realize, is that in every case I had a choice. Once I went to the edges of my own personal hell and back, everything was colored by that experience.

It helped that I had a natural tendency to live in the moment. For me, it was a natural way to see the world. It's not that I wouldn't worry. It's just that I never allowed that worry to impede my exuberance for life. The obvious limitations provided easy excuses for negativity and self-doubt. The greater challenge would be to assert my freedom and individuality through positive actions. Rather than wallow in reasons for not making the most of my life, I looked only to ways I could give further meaning to my life. I was excited about what was coming next rather than anxious about the future or despondent about the past. To this day, that approach helps me navigate the world. Only now I have to do it differently.

My support structure contributed to my worldview, particularly when I came home. I emerged from a year in the hospital unable to move, but it was and continues to be a non-issue. I was barely twenty years old when I left rehab. It was as if I had been teleported from a reckless life on and off the football field. I might as well have been abducted by aliens and probed for an entire year, then suddenly returned with a reconstituted perspective and a clean slate to begin a new phase in my life's journey.

Certainly there were adjustments, though mine were relatively easy compared to others less fortunate. My family was able to avoid the crushing financial demands attendant to most catastrophic injuries. The vast majority of people in my condition don't have insurance sufficient to cover the medical costs, much less the financial resources to make a house wheelchair-accessible, or buy a customized van, a power wheelchair, and the ongoing and neverending cost of quality care. The fact that my father worked for U.S. Tobacco probably saved my life. The firm's catastrophic insurance policy covered the vast majority of bills and afforded me the very best medical care at a cost in the tens of millions of dollars.

To be sure, the costs associated with caring for a quadriplegic are staggering. Even for people fortunate enough to have insurance, the financial stress can be nearly as devastating to a family as the actual injury. Most policies reach lifetime limits within the first few months of care. The entire family becomes physically and emotionally paralyzed by the extreme economic burdens. Families, even those with savings, can be drained within months. Usually, someone in the family, a mother, brother, or sister, eventually is forced to suspend his or her life to care for the injured person. At that point, everyone is in survival mode, which is hard to sustain over time.

The cost of private nurses is upwards of $500,000 a year. My wheelchair and van alone cost a combined $100,000. Then there are the medications, numerous medical supplies unique to someone in my condition, doctors visits, transportation costs, and occasional hospitalizations. That doesn't include the fact that my home has to be completely accessible. All told it costs $1 million a year to keep me healthy and moving. A medical emergency that results in extended hospitalization could double or triple that number. That's the problem with a catastrophic injury: It never stops being catastrophic.

That's why I never look back. I never ask, "Why me?" I recognize I am fortunate. I am not going to waste another chance at enjoying life. That's why I wanted to finish college. No one had to talk me into it. No one expected me to go back to school. I knew the idea of getting a degree was important to my mom, but school had become important to me.

For the first time in my life, I had a desire to be in school. I wanted to learn. There was apprehension but it was outweighed by excitement. I took a tour of the University of Miami campus. It was an eye-opening experience to say the least. I went to an all-boys high school, followed by the all-male college life at The Citadel. After traveling through the halls of UM and seeing one beautiful girl after another, I only had one thought: "Sign me up!" I really did want to learn, but the scenery helped seal the deal.

The most difficult part of going to school was getting admitted. Once my grades were transferred from The Citadel, Miami put me on automatic probation. I was told, very clearly, "You have to earn a minimum grade average of 2.5 the first semester or you're out."

There weren't many people going to college in wheelchairs in the mid-1980s. I decided to take it one semester at a time. I signed up for two classes—public relations and marketing.

Fran Matera taught the first class I took at UM. She was very attractive and kind enough to give me a tour of the Communications Department. I attended class like any other student. Only I was in a wheelchair and traveled with a nurse. I still played the angles. Basically, I asked the cutest girl in the class to share her notes with me. After class, I'd get the notes photocopied, take her to lunch, and use that opportunity to flirt. Of course, I always preferred the most attractive girl. But just to be safe, and probably for the first time in my educational career, I made sure that I was prepared. Sometimes it meant I had two or more sets of notes. That's because sometimes the prettiest girl wasn't the most studious. I never missed a class at the University of Miami.

I read all the material. I actually studied. The education process was straightforward, except for taking tests. It was a normal college experience. In fact, it was far more normal compared to college life at The Citadel.

Tests separated me from regular students. If we had a multiple-choice test, then I had to take it either before or after class. Some tests were oral, just the teacher and me. As a result, I had to know the material, which was a departure from all prior school experience. Before, I was essentially a professional cheater and generally indifferent to rituals of schooling. Now I was on my own. There were no cheat sheets and not a trick in the book that would help me.

It wasn't until I attended the University of Miami that I learned how to write, the hard way. I realized how far behind I was compared to other students. The computer technology was a long way from where it is today. I typed papers using a "mouth stick," which looks exactly like it sounds. I had to punch one letter at a time. Writing a paper took me forever. I always had a nurse with me, but I never asked anyone to help me type. I didn't even ask them to turn the page of a book. I'd use the mouth stick instead.

School started clicking right away. I earned a 3.5 grade-point-average that first semester. For the first time in my life, I was excited to bring home my report card. After all the years of manipulating the system and doing everything possible to avoid the inevitable stress that accompanied every previous report card, I couldn't wait to show my mother. Of course, typical of my mother, the success only confirmed her suspicions.

"I knew it! I knew you could do it all along."

My mom was right. I could have been a much better student. If I had given as much effort in school as I did trying to avoid it, then I wouldn't have been so unprepared. I always knew I was smarter than my performance suggested. Only now I was making a determined effort. It wasn't until I took a second-semester English class that I realized just how unprepared and behind I was. It took me until my twenty-first year of life to learn how to compose a grammatically correct sentence and to care whether or not I could.

I realized that I couldn't rely on my body anymore. Until my injury, I always thought that sports, football in particular, would take me everywhere I needed to go. One of the greatest ironies of my injury, from the perspective of friends, was the fact that I had always been known as the most active among us. I was the first to start a game of Frisbee or football at the beach. I never stood still. Now I had to start using my brain because that's all I had.

It was a radical transformation. At the same time, I had to redirect my passion and spirit for life. I recognized the opportunity and understood the concept—dare for greatness. Everything I had accomplished previously was done physically. Now I had to do everything on the basis of heart. We don't necessarily know what's inside of us, or what we are capable of. In my case, what was inside me had been hidden by the physical actions that dominated my life. Now I was forced to find another way.

Everything in my life was forced to operate at a much slower pace. In many respects, it was a welcome change from the high-velocity, high-intensity, high-risk lifestyle of my youth.

I acquired a new asset: patience.

* * *

DAD: The real question was: How was Marc going to go back to school?

It wasn't a question of finances. Rather, how was he physically going to handle the course load, the logistical problems, and manage schoolwork that had to be done at home?

This was a kid who had been totally negligent with regard to academics. His thought processes had been anything but academic. So when he wanted to go back to school, I was very proud of him. But I also figured that, with most things Marc did to that point in his life, it wouldn't last long, especially with the additional burden of the wheelchair.

I knew every test had to be oral, which meant he had to know the material. I thought it would be a very difficult process for him. Then we found out that after all those years of fighting the education system, he decided that he really did want to use his brain.

Marc spent more than a year in the hospital. For the most part, he was unable to communicate freely. He had a lot of time to think and reflect. The first two or three months he was home, he didn't watch television or do much of anything.

The point is that when Marc made the decision to go back to school it wasn't a spur-of-the-moment decision.

Chapter 46

The Gospel According to Bob

I was drawn to the Rastafarian philosophy back in high school. I fell in love with the music when I heard Rita Marley's song "One Draw." You hear people talk about how a particular piece of music "spoke" to them. Well, that's what happened to me with reggae music. And, aligned with the melodies and lyrics, the abiding philosophy of live and let live resonated with my then-immature and shortsighted interpretation of its key tenets. So, too, did the social preoccupation with smoking pot and gliding with the wind rather than swimming against the current.

At the University of Miami, I started hanging out with an old high school friend, Johnny Guardiola (a.k.a. Johnny Dread). A Bob Marley CD blaring on my car speakers in the Columbus parking lot sparked our friendship. We made an instant connection.

Johnny played the drums. He hooked up with Bob Marley's step-brother, Anthony Booker, and another musician named Bagga. The three of them were performing gigs throughout South Florida, and I would often join them. Bagga was extremely talented. He played just about every instrument. He also was an excellent mentor to Johnny and Anthony. Johnny didn't have the best natural ability, but he made up for it with hard work and passion. Our relationship evolved from just hanging out to an immersion into the music and its culture. Eventually the friendship led to a sound studio and the creation of a record label.

I recognized that the music business was only slightly less risky than the lottery. But I loved the music and these guys were attracting a nice following. At the time, we had another friend who was recording at the Miami Sound Studio, the place where Gloria Estefan got her start. The owner and engineer, Carlos Diaz Granados, always had money issues. One day he made me an offer.

"Listen man, for $1,000 I'll let you record as long as you want to come up with a single."

Within twenty-four hours, Marcus Records was born, and I was in the music business. The idea was to make a record, then see where I could take it. Once a week, we'd head into the studio and work on songs. We weren't sure which song to lay down. Then one day Carlos called me with an even better offer.

"I've got a better deal for you, Marc. For $5,000 I'll give you one night a week for as long as you want so you can make an entire album. I'll do all the engineering and editing."

Johnny, Bagga, and a few other guys came together and we formed a band, Copacetic. We recorded every Thursday night. I even brought my dad and his college roommate, Uncle Rich, a musician himself, to the studio one night. It was a lot of fun. I couldn't learn enough about the business.

After about a year of work, we laid down ten really good songs and produced an album, *Ghetto Rock*. I shopped it all over the country. I was able to get distribution in South Florida and throughout the Southeast. The album made it into the Top 10 on the World Music charts.

Then band woes emerged. It was the same old rock and roll story. Infighting and greed devolved into a dysfunctional atmosphere. Eventually I became fed up. I was getting calls every day that one guy or another needed money.

At the time the band was doing pretty well touring up and down the East Coast. We released the album in 1990, and we opened up for well-known bands such as Third World and The Wailers. Ziggy Marley performed with Copacetic in several live shows. On the first Sunday of every month we headlined at Woody's on the Beach, a club owned by the Rolling Stones guitarist Ronnie Wood. The band was making a name for itself, and it showed in album sales and at events. There were some positive articles written about the band, too, including a great write-up in the College Music Journal.

Then Hurricane Andrew blew it all away.

I had moved my office down south to Cutler Ridge, a city south of Miami. I was sharing a warehouse with a good friend, Steve Petrillo, whom I was helping with his business. All the records were stored at the warehouse when Andrew hit South Florida.

I happened to be in New York with Steve at a celebrity golf tournament. My parents told me to stay in New York until the hurricane passed. No one imagined the extent of the devastation to come. The next morning, August 25, 1992, I called all over South Florida. There was no phone service. The television stations didn't have reporters on the scene yet, so it wasn't immediately clear how bad things were.

We called a friend at the CBS affiliate in Tampa. He said, "You guys are OK. It didn't hit Miami directly. It hit a place called 'something dale.'" The answer confused Steve and me.

"What do you mean, 'something dale?' Do you mean Hallandale?"

"No."

"Fort Lauderdale?"

"No. It's something like Ken Dale."

Then it hit me. He meant Kendall, which was my neighborhood. Steve and I had the same thought:

"Oh my God!"

We needed to get home. My van was at Miami International. The closest operational airport was West Palm Beach, which is about seventy miles north. We arrived around six or seven that night, rented a car, and headed south down I-95. By then I had been in contact with my parents, who were fine. Steve couldn't get in touch with anyone, so we decided to go to his house first, which was located in Redland, a farming community south of Miami. As we drove down the highway, nothing seemed particularly out of the ordinary until we approached

SW 152nd Street. That turned out to be the demarcation zone where the northern wall of the storm passed.

As we exited the highway, there was a car dealership, completely demolished. We turned down that street, and there were fifty- to sixty-foot-tall cement telephone poles down all over. That meant anyone trying to drive on that road either couldn't pass, or had to create a new road, which they did. These new roadways went through people's backyards, fields, and anywhere a vehicle could navigate.

Frames of houses and all sorts of debris were scattered everywhere. It wasn't easy finding our way. Nothing was familiar because all of the usual landmarks were gone. Steve lived on a farm down a dirt road. To reach his house we had to stop the car so he could get out and, literally, climb over and through trees. There were a hundred pine trees on his property. All of them were blown down. He had to be one of the luckiest people on Earth because not one of them fell on his house, which had only one broken window despite the fact that virtually every house around his was destroyed.

From there we drove to my parents' house. Coral Gables was generally untouched, but there were trees down everywhere. To navigate the neighborhood, we had to drive on the golf course, behind houses. I recognized the street, but I had to figure out how to get from the street to the house due to all the downed trees. My parents rode out the storm at home because Coral Gables wasn't in the path of the storm. But the power was out everywhere. I had to go to The Miami Project every day for three weeks just to recharge my wheelchair. That meant cold showers, spotty phone service, and no air-conditioning in ninety-five-degree Miami heat.

All things considered, I had nothing to complain about. Andrew destroyed lives and changed an entire region. Many rebuilt while others moved north to start a new life in Broward and Palm Beach counties, and beyond. Amid the devastation and its aftermath, Andrew revealed the courage and compassion of a large and diverse community.

Ultimately, Andrew blew away Marcus Records. An ill wind was blowing around the business anyway, so it was time. But this had been my first attempt at a significant venture in my new life. Therefore, the music business provided an invaluable experience and life lesson. For that reason alone, the experience was a success.

I had proven to myself that I could aspire to and achieve a goal beyond the bounds of my former physical identity.

Now it was time to move forward once more.

* * *

DAD: It took Marc's injury for him to find the time to reflect on his life and where it was going. Only then do I think that the lifestyle Terry and I gave the kids became part of his life.

All of a sudden, those basic ethics of hard work and respect hit home with Marc. If he hadn't been injured, he might not have slowed down. I think eventually he would have been OK. I think he would have done very well. But I also think he would have had bumps in the road because he would have exhausted his wild side before he was ready to accept the responsibilities in front of him. It might have resulted in him being arrested or some other kind of trouble.

Marc got through the early days of his injury not with God but through the Rastafarian philosophy of life. He loved the music, he smoked grass, and he did all the things that he thought were going to help him get through life in a chair. He had many rough patches.

Still, his mind was working 100 percent of the time. He put together a record label. He put together a group. Marc was willing to fund and drive the business. The only reason it didn't become as successful as it might have is because the guys didn't share Marc's commitment. Marc told them he was giving them one more shot to show up for rehearsal. They didn't show up. So Marc disbanded the business.

He spent a year working on the band and putting the infrastructure in place for the label. Then he did what he had to do. It's exactly the same thing I would have done. I wouldn't have tolerated those guys not show-ing up to work.

Chapter 47

The Psychology of Me

Every once in a while, I'd meet up with Father Roger Radloff, a Catholic priest who served as the psychologist for other clergy within the Archdiocese of Miami. He was a Jungian analyst—a graduate of the prestigious C.G. Jung Institute in Zurich, Switzerland.

I hadn't seen Roger, whom my mother referred to as the "family shrink," since I was in eighth grade. I was terrorizing my mother, ignoring schoolwork, and avoiding responsibilities. As my mother tells the story, at such a young age, I didn't seem to be getting any-thing out of the counseling sessions so she started going instead. Eventually, Roger became a good friend and an important mentor.

After my injury I visited him regularly, in a kind of informal manner, not as a patient, just to talk. Although a Catholic priest, he was perhaps the most open-minded individual I have ever known. He was a great listener, never judgmental, and uncannily wise. Roger provided a venue to reveal my thoughts and feelings about the entirely new life in which I found myself. I had endured the emotional spec-trum. In his unique way he helped me understand, appreciate, and come to terms with my many questions. Those included the funda-mental questions about the nature of God—a God who would allow pain and suffering—and the purpose of religion.

During my first couple of semesters at the University of Miami, I was just a kid in college. At the start of my second year, I switched from Communications to Business. That didn't last long. I was taking economics and accounting courses, neither of which was my strong subject, being that they required hands-on math. I literally couldn't do it. Those kinds of courses were out of my realm and beyond the available technology. I wasn't inspired by those disciplines either. More and more I found myself looking for an area of study with which I could identify directly—something that would speak to me.

One day I was talking to Roger, and it just clicked. Psychology was the perfect subject matter because it had direct application to my life. Not only could it help me understand my situation, but psychology could inform and facilitate my interactions with others. Even then, a big part of my day was providing support to families and individuals dealing with spinal cord injuries through The Miami Project.

Studying the mind and human behavior better prepared me to understand what people were experiencing psychologically and emotionally. My studies became an invaluable tool that I use in my private and public lives. I became an ambassador for The Miami Project and a perpetual advocate for the disabled community.

Chapter 48

An Away Game at The Citadel

When my father first mentioned filing a lawsuit against The Citadel, the news came and went without a second thought. It was a couple months after my injury. I was still fighting for my life. I couldn't care less about a lawsuit. I remember telling my father to do what he needed to do. It was fine with me. Starting in the fall of 1985 and into 1986 we filed a lawsuit against The Citadel, the team trainer, Andy Clausen, and the team doctor, E.K. Wallace.

It wasn't until I was transferred from the hospital to the rehabilitation center that the enormity of the situation became clear as lawyers took my deposition. I understood the position my father and the lawyers were taking. I had no reason to believe that The Citadel would not support me as one of its fallen. Instead, the school turned everything over to lawyers. It was the cold lack of concern for anything but their liability that so bothered my father. I didn't disagree, but I still felt uncomfortable about filing the suit. I understood the rationale; it just didn't feel right. I knew the trial would force my classmates and teammates to take sides.

When I returned for my class's graduation in 1988, I didn't feel welcomed by the administration. They definitely didn't roll out any red carpet. There was a tension in the air, like two boxers eyeing each other

before a bout. The only thing that was important to me was being there
to recognize my classmates and teammates. Some of those guys had
become really good friends, but my injury and the subsequent legal
battle tested that friendship.

Once the lawsuit was filed, The Citadel went on lockdown. Citadel officials sat down with the entire team to inform them of our suit.
They told the players that no one was to talk to anyone about me, or
the injury, without first notifying the coaches and/or the administration. Our lawyers eventually deposed every player on the team. The
net result was that I had teammates testifying against me. What did
they testify to? Essentially that I hit too hard. One of them went so far
as to say that I intentionally tried to hurt people on the field. I had to
read all the depositions to note any discrepancies or mistakes so that I
could alert our lawyers. I read at least fifty depositions. Some of them
were very difficult for me to read. Among them were the statements
of young men who played on my defensive team and for whom I had
great respect. Of course, there also were those who testified on my
behalf.

Our lawyers knew I would be attending my class's graduation ceremony. They instructed me to show no emotion.

"Don't smile, don't say anything," they admonished.

Colonel Harvey Dick was the Commandant of Cadets. He was
responsible for carrying out disciplinary actions. First and foremost,
he was someone to be feared. Just the sound of his voice commanded
respect. He was tough, but he was also fair. During my time at The
Citadel, Colonel Dick and I had created a friendship and bond forged
by mutual respect. He walked over to say hello. He was being nice,
telling jokes. But I didn't even crack a smile.

"What's wrong, Buoniconti? Can't smile?"

"No Colonel, I can't."

It was tough being there. I could feel the tension. But it was important for me to be there for my teammates and classmates, especially
my company-mates from F-Troop. It was those individuals in particular with whom I felt a bond no one else could possibly understand.
No circumstance could dissolve that connection. We spent our entire
freshman year relying on one another just to make it through the day

full of countless inspections, marching, physical and verbal abuse, and every rule and procedure that tested our resolve. As a demonstration of their loyalty, in their senior year my company-mates, following a longstanding Citadel tradition, painted my name alongside theirs on the steps of the four-story spiral staircase—something only reserved for those few who had made it that far. It was the ultimate expression of what my time with them meant. My name on the step symbolized the bond that allowed us to survive our knob year. That bond kept my spirit present to them, even in my absence, and through the rest of our lives.

A couple months later, in the summer of 1988, I returned to Charleston for the trial. As I said, I felt uneasy about the entire process. I didn't feel good about the fact we were suing the school and the trainer.

The media were everywhere when the trial started. I was in court every day for the six-week trial. I told our lawyers that I shouldn't be there at all, other than when I had to testify. But they insisted that my presence was essential in order to alert them to any discrepancies during the proceedings. The trial was emotionally draining for everyone in my family, especially my mom. One of the first people to testify was my teammate and friend John Stephens. My dad testified too, as did several doctors, including Dr. Charles Virgin, the former physician to the Miami Dolphins, and Dr. Green. We even had Dick Butkus, the Hall of Fame Chicago Bears linebacker, testify as an expert witness, with respect to the legality—the mechanics—of my tackle.

The defense lawyers argued that I had "speared" Herman Jacobs, the running back. That is, that I had intentionally used the top of my helmet in making the tackle, which would have constituted an illegal hit. Butkus said it was a legal tackle. So did the referee, who was standing right over the play when it happened. I saw that same referee fifteen years later working a Dolphins game. I was on the sidelines in my wheelchair when he came over and said, "Marc, you probably don't remember me, but I was the referee in the game you were injured. I testified on your behalf at the trial. I just want you to know that to this day I believe you made a clean tackle."

He had no idea how important those few words were to me. Admittedly, I tried to hurt other players throughout my career. It wasn't like the alleged New Orleans Saints bounty scandal where players and coaches were offered money for targeting opponents. But football is like war. It gets ugly. Players try to impose their will on the opposition. Those moments and those experiences are like walking on hallowed ground. To this day, and I'm sure for the rest of my life, I will cherish my football memories. I'll never forget the battles fought together as a team.

I knew in my heart that on that play, I was just doing my best to make the tackle, with no animosity or ill intentions. I always prided myself as a leader on the field. I knew proper tackling technique. I strived to make it as perfect as possible. In the end, I knew that on that play, on that day, I executed according to the rules of the game. I did it right.

One of the stories our lawyers told was of an injury to my leg during the season. I went to the infirmary without telling my coaches. The next day, the coaches pulled me aside and worked me out for two hours. Their point: Don't ever fake an injury and try to get a day off by not telling the coaching staff.

I wasn't faking anything, but that didn't matter. The coaches made their point loud and clear. My lawyers used that experience in the trial:

"Marc was scared. He didn't want to show how injured he was because he had experienced firsthand what could happen. They punished players for being injured."

After we had presented our case, The Citadel offered to settle. The school had a $1 million insurance policy, so we took their $800,000 offer. As a result, halfway through the trial The Citadel was no longer a part of the case.

The rest of the trial was against Dr. Wallace. When he got up on the stand the discrepancies in his testimony were unbelievable. I had people tell me that there was no way we were going to lose after the doctor's performance. Our lawyers tore him apart. When it was all said and done, the jury only took a few hours. In the deliberations there was screaming by members of the jury, but whoever did the yelling apparently didn't scream loudly enough on my behalf. When the jury reconvened my lawyer said, "It doesn't look good." When the not guilty verdict was announced, I wanted to leave as quickly as possible. The next morning, I was gone.

It's safe to say the jury might have been somewhat swayed in the home team's favor. There were undoubtedly jurors who thought that the Buonicontis didn't need the money and that whatever money we would receive would be leaving the great state of South Carolina. Their lawyers put up a good defense. Our lawyers made a heck of a case, too, but it was complicated.

I recall someone telling me that I was part of the problem in making our case. "You looked too good," he said. "You were healthy enough to sit through eight-hour days in a courtroom. Ironically, your presence, even in a wheelchair, was a negative."

* * *

DAD: I made sure I was at the trial 95 percent of the time. There was certain testimony that I felt I had to be present for. I had responsibilities to my company and its shareholders. It was hard going back and forth, but when I needed to be there, I found a way.

Our representation was good, but we had to overcome the prejudice of the colloquial neighborhood of South Carolina.

What are you going to appeal? It was a jury listening to the facts. They came to a verdict. I don't know whether we could have appealed on the basis of a technicality or not.

Had The Citadel simply supported Marc, and told us, "Don't worry about it. We're going to take care of things. He's one of our soldiers. We don't leave anyone alone on the battlefield," then we probably wouldn't have sued.

All they had to do in my mind was to recognize the fact that Marc went into the game as one of their men. That's not asking much. They were worried about a lawsuit more than they were concerned about the welfare of one of their soldiers.

Chapter 49

I'm No Doctor

I had two epiphanies during my last year in college. Eleven years after my injury, I had become so invested in school that I started down the path toward my doctorate. It wasn't an easy decision because the academic demands meant I wouldn't have as much time to commit to The Miami Project. I knew that was an issue for my colleagues. It was an internal struggle. I felt a sense of guilt for wanting to pursue a personal goal at the expense of investing even more time on behalf of finding a cure.

The first epiphany was prompted by an experience in my first graduate-level course in psychology. The class convened at the professor's home, which was exactly the kind of off-center approach to life that I appreciated. I went to the house with enthusiasm. Other students were already waiting just inside the doorway, gathered together in a small library.

The professor appeared from upstairs. "Alright, let's go upstairs."

Without hesitation every student followed the professor's lead and headed up the stairs. I was left sitting in the foyer. There was no way for me to get my wheelchair to where the class was going to take place. No one seemed to notice.

"Oh, can you hear from down there?" the professor uttered from the room above.

"Yeah, sure."

I was stunned. The guy proceeded to teach the class without a second thought. I wasn't sure what to say because I was so shocked. If that happened today, I would let him know exactly what I thought of his insensitivity. Needless to say, I didn't feel as though I was part of the class.

It's telling the way many people unconsciously expressed their attitudes towards the disabled. It was as if the assumption of the day was that a disability excluded you from the social norms and expectations. Back then a wheelchair was a convenient excuse to absolve one of engaging on a personal and intimate level. We were seen as not only different, but something less compared to everyone else.

To prove a point, I brought an eight-foot piece of plywood to the next class. I had my nurse lay it on the professor's stairs so I could drive my wheelchair right into his house. By then the entire experience had turned me off. I thought, "I can continue going to school, attending classes and listening to lectures, or I can channel my energies into something with a meaningful purpose." I continued to participate in the class. I did what I had to do. Ironically, it was while working on a paper for that class that I had my second epiphany.

I was at home writing on my computer. Suddenly, I had an overwhelming urge to urinate. Usually I would urinate on my own and without the assistance of a nurse. This time I could feel my bladder contracting with spasms. I knew something was wrong. I called my nurse and asked him to catheterize me.

At the time I'd have it done twice a day, once in the morning and once at night. The process is straightforward. The nurse takes a tube and inserts it through my urethra into the bladder so that it drains. This time, though, he couldn't get the tube into my bladder. The tubes are called "red rubber catheters" and they aren't very rigid. My nurse kept pushing the tube forward, but my sphincter muscles were locked. He couldn't force the tube into the bladder, which meant the urine couldn't be released.

What happened next is called autonomic dysreflexia. It manifests itself differently depending on the circumstances. The bladder might be full, the person might be sitting incorrectly, or something noxious could be affecting the body. It doesn't matter whether it's a broken bone, a blood clot, a hangnail, or an infection. Because I don't feel a pain sensation, my body sends a different kind of stimulus. In other words, my autonomic system starts to react.

When I couldn't urinate, despite the intense pressure built up, I started sweating. My skin became clammy. My veins and arteries began to constrict, which rapidly increased my heart rate and blood pressure. I couldn't urinate for an hour. My body was responding wildly. We tried three or four times to get the tube into my bladder and all the while I was sweating profusely. My heart rate continued to climb. The immediate danger is a stroke, which is not uncommon under those circumstances.

I started to panic. Thankfully, my mother lived next door. We were about to call 911, when I asked the nurse to try one more time. This time, he was able to push the tube into my bladder. There was so much pressure that, when released, urine sprayed ten feet across the room. The feeling was so intense that I was crying like a baby in the arms of my mom. After about ten minutes, all the symptoms dissipated. It was a powerful reminder of the fragility and precariousness of my life—how in an instant I could be faced with a life-threatening emergency.

By the next day, I had a massive urinary tract infection, and I was back in the hospital. The experience woke me up. It was yet another reminder of my mortality. Although I seemed to be living a relatively normal life on the surface, I was actually navigating a precipice while holding a ticking time bomb.

All of this occurred right around the time my parents were going through their divorce, so it was quite an emotional time.

To understand my parents' relationship, you have to remember that they had been high school sweethearts. My mom knew my father before the fame that came with a Hall of Fame professional football career, or before he became a business tycoon and a media celebrity. They were kids. They never lost sight of where they had come from.

The bright lights and glamour that surrounded my father amounted to nothing more than a flicker to my mom.

As his popularity grew, my mom was still that old-fashioned girl from Springfield with whom my father had fallen in love. In my mom's mind, nothing had changed. But everything had changed around my father. That disconnect, between the past and the present, eventually manifested. My dad was spending more and more time in New York and Connecticut. His career at UST kept evolving upward, and he remained a sports celebrity due to his HBO show.

But when my dad came home, he was just that old-fashioned boy from Springfield my mother had fallen in love with. Outside of our house, it was bright lights and cheers. When my dad came home, he was a father and a husband. Instead of a standing ovation, my mother might say, "Take out of the garbage."

Like all relationships that fall out of sync, no matter how much love is involved, there comes a time to acknowledge that both would be better off going their separate ways. Regardless of the personal differences, when it came to family nothing changed. My parents' commitment, bond, and love remained resolute.

When I left the hospital a few days later, I realized how selfish it was for me to pursue a doctorate. I recognized I had a larger responsibility to The Project—one that was well beyond any personal goal I might have for myself. I also realized I had no desire to be asked by an insensitive, self-absorbed teacher if I was "OK" while sitting alone in the entryway of his house. I actually called the guy from the hospital to let him know I wouldn't be in class. He never even returned the call.

In a way, I'm glad it worked out the way it did. Earning a doctorate would have been a nice personal achievement, but there was more to be done outside of school. Once more, the lesson came through loud and clear: Life is too short. And it's shorter still for me. I needed to do the right thing. That meant focusing my life on finding a cure.

Chapter 50

Balancing a Life on the Edge

I was a kid when I was injured. It took surviving a catastrophic injury and life in a wheelchair to shape me into a man. I wouldn't say it's been a smooth process. It certainly presented unprecedented challenges.

On one hand, I was enjoying life. I earned a college degree, traveled and hung out with my friends, pursued all kinds of interests, and supported all of my father's hard work on behalf of The Miami Project. I also had some remarkable experiences that probably wouldn't have been available to me had I not been injured. President George H. W. Bush appointed me to his Points of Light Foundation. Sen. Jack Kemp, then Secretary of Housing and Urban Development, named me to the HUD Committee for the Disabled. I received the Jefferson Award for Public Service at the White House. I interacted with President Bill Clinton, and President Richard Nixon, a giving man who went out of his way to personally help The Miami Project.

The flip side of that coin, however, was much darker and never far enough in the distance.

I was having severe bacterial infections in my urological system that had become resistant to a host of antibiotics. I was in and out of the hospital. I had various surgical procedures to remove kidney stones. Still, I kept getting infections.

Unlike a normal urinary tract system that produces urine in the kidneys and drains into the bladder, a neurogenic bladder like mine doesn't have functional control. My bladder and kidneys are fine. It's the emptying process that causes problems and leads to the infections. The controlling muscle, called the sphincter, doesn't work. If I get too much urine in the bladder, then it can leak, or back up into my kidneys, causing renal failure. I am prone to infection because I can't empty my bladder properly.

What makes it all the more distressing is that it happens without warning. I have to look at my urine to see whether it's cloudy, or has a distinctive smell that indicates an infection. I had septicemia once, a condition where the bacteria were so prolific that they moved into my bloodstream. Even a healthy person without my complications can die quite easily from becoming septic. In one instance, I was in the admitting department at the hospital when I suddenly couldn't see straight. I could see only half of everything even with both eyes open. I couldn't comprehend or respond to questions. I was confused for a couple days after that incident. It was a close call.

By 1996, more than a decade after my initial injury, I was constantly going into the hospital for heavy doses of antibiotics to kill the bacteria building up in my bladder. A month later, the infection would be back again. The bacteria were hiding in kidney stones, another common problem for people like me. The antibiotics couldn't penetrate the stones. As soon as I stopped taking the drugs, the bacteria came out of the stones and into my system. Eventually, I had to get all the stones removed.

Quadriplegics maintain a precarious balance between sickness and health, life and death. Any one of ten things could kill me on any given day. It's like walking in a minefield. You don't know which step is going to kill you. Navigation comes down to knowing your body as thoroughly as possible. Often even that's not enough. I woke one day coughing up blood. A little later I coughed up another clot of blood. Back to the hospital, another series of tests. This time I had a blood clot in my leg, parts of which had traveled into my lungs, where it became a pulmonary embolism. Few things can kill a person faster and without notice than an embolism. Again, it's particularly problematic for someone with paralysis because the circulatory system is compromised by a sedentary lifestyle. One high-profile victim of an embolism was former NFL great Derrick Thomas, who died as a result of complications from an embolism shortly after being paralyzed in a car accident.

In addition to my physical challenges, we had setbacks at The Miami Project as well, though not through any lack of effort by my father. We knew that the kind of research necessary to truly make a difference required a much deeper financial commitment. We needed our own building so that we could attract the world's top researchers and doctors.

Chapter 51

The Buoniconti Fund

In the days and weeks following my injury a reality set in. It wasn't just that there was nothing anyone could do. There was hardly anyone in the world even making an effort. That fact was disorienting for my father.

When Dr. Green introduced the idea of The Miami Project to Cure Paralysis it was like flipping a light switch.

My father has always controlled his own destiny. He is self-reliant, relentless when necessary, and always operating on his own terms. There was nothing he could do about what happened to me. As a result, my father lost his center. He needed to find meaning amid the wreckage. The Miami Project presented an opportunity, even if it came with apparently insurmountable challenges. Then my dad did what he always did. He used every ounce of energy he had to get the job done.

"Is there anything going on with spinal cord injury research that provides hope?"

Dr. Green, long frustrated by a hardened scientific consensus, had a simple answer: "No."

The Jackson Health System is a public trust. The trust, in partnership with the University of Miami Miller School of Medicine, agreed in the spring of 1986 to support The Miami Project. The idea was to bring together the greatest research minds from around the world in the spirit of the Manhattan Project or NASA. It was a considerable leap of faith given the scientific consensus.

The scientific community thought the name—The Miami Project to Cure Paralysis—created false hope. Scientists called Dr. Green crazy and warned that the endeavor to find a cure was way too ambitious. After all, the spinal cord is a very inhospitable environment. Cells effectively kill themselves at the site of an injury.

The facts were a perfect set up for people like Dr. Green and my dad. They would find the money to change the paradigm. From their perspective, the science was an obstacle to be overcome. The negative sentiment by the establishment was galling, but from the beginning it fueled the effort.

A world-class board was assembled to find a scientific director. Fundraising commenced, driven by people who had far more passion than experience.

Jack Schneider, managing partner of Allen & Company, was a family friend. He suggested a fundraising event in New York City honoring the world's greatest athletes. Don Misner and Beth Roscoe, both paralyzed patients of Dr. Green's, helped a small team of people organize multiple initiatives at the outset. In the first few years of The Great Sports Legend dinner, we honored some of the biggest names in the history of sports—Joe DiMaggio, Muhammad Ali, A.J. Foyt, Red Auerbach, Arthur Ashe, Sugar Ray Leonard, Joe Namath, Bobby Orr, Mario Andretti, Gordie Howe, Stan Musial, Floyd Patterson, Johnny Unitas, Frank Gifford, Bobby Hull, and Mickey Mantle to name a handful.

President Richard Nixon called to volunteer his support. Mr. Nixon was a big football fan. He had a house on Biscayne Bay and spent a lot of time in Florida, even as president. He loved my father. When President Nixon was still in the White House and the Dolphins were at the height of their greatness, the president named two Vietnam War bombing missions "Operation Linebacker" and "Operation Linebacker II." I have no idea whether the success of my father and the Dolphins influenced his choices, but President Nixon was that kind of fan.

He was also a fan of The Miami Project. President Nixon dedicated our first clinical research program, called "The Bantle Center," named in honor of Lou Bantle, who was chairman of U.S. Tobacco.

By the time I left the hospital for good in late 1986, a worldwide search had produced The Miami Project's first scientific director, Dr. Åke Sager. Dr. Sager was an up-and-coming neurologist and a leading scientist in the field of paralysis at Sweden's acclaimed Karolinska Institute. It was critical to attract a scientist with Dr. Sager's international name recognition. His arrival put The Miami Project on the map, though not without controversy. An article in the (Fort Lauderdale) *SunSentinel* criticized The Miami Project for attempting to do the impossible—cure paralysis. Left unsaid was the obvious. Every scientific breakthrough is impossible if no one is making an effort.

The criticism affected Dr. Sager the same way it affected my dad. They just worked harder. Dr. Sager's work revolved around cell regeneration. The objective was to understand how cells in the spinal cord function after an injury, then design methodologies either to change the environment around the injury or to promote transplant strategies for regeneration. The science was oriented toward improving the quality of life of paralyzed people by improving function.

The Miami Project's first-year budget was one million dollars, and every dollar of it had to be raised. The organization grew quickly though. Then, in 1989, Dr. Sager was offered the chair of the neurology department at the Karolinska Institute. It was an offer he couldn't refuse, and Dr. Sager returned to Sweden. This time our search came with some cachet and a promise.

The global neuroscience community took notice when the husband-wife team of Dr. Richard Bunge and Dr. Mary Bunge joined The Miami Project. Richard was named scientific director in 1989. Their research suggested an eventual change to the scientific paradigm. Dr. Green also promised them that The Miami Project would find the money, talent, and space to take their life's work to human trials. The Bunges were doing leading-edge work with Schwann cells, peripheral nerve cells that showed unusual potential for regeneration.

The process of attracting such high-profile scientists was not unlike recruiting five-star football players at a major university. We needed to prove to them that we had the facilities, the culture, and the resources to build a world-class team. The Bunges brought at least ten scientists with them. Our budget grew to $5 million a year.

It's important to note that, unlike well-established conditions such as diabetes, heart and lung diseases, and cancer, there was no fund-raising infrastructure for spinal cord injury research. The population of paralyzed people is quite small compared to chronic diseases that affect millions. All of which made fundraising infinitely more difficult, particularly at the speed at which The Miami Project was growing.

Within a couple years, we were housed in seven different buildings. The science was progressing, but we needed more space. We also needed to expand our horizons. The Buoniconti Fund was incorporated as a 501(c)(3) nonprofit on January 31, 1991. First, we needed to expand our geographical and logistical reach beyond Miami. Second, we needed flexibility. Working with Jackson and the University of Miami is great, but there is a formal bureaucratic decision-making process that comes with public and private institutions. Third, we needed a substantial amount of money in order to build a world-class research facility.

As president of a major tobacco company, my dad spent a lot of time in Washington, DC. He also had a lot of friends on the Hill, including then-Speaker of the House Tip O'Neill. Mr. O'Neill listened to my dad's pitch, and promised to walk him through the process of raising public money to build a separate research building.

With Mr. O'Neill clearing the way, my dad tirelessly worked the halls of Congress. He met with members of Congress, senators, and entire committees. In March 1992, a formal request for proposal (RFP) was issued for the construction of an $18 million neuroscience center. The RFP was written in a way that favored The Miami Project's unique attributes. We responded to the RFP a month later, and the award was scheduled for the summer. Though not quite a formality, everyone involved was confident of a positive resolution.

On the day of the award, my dad was sitting in a board meeting of the Jackson Public Trust. He excused himself and went outside to hear the news.

At the last minute, our very own senator had intervened on behalf of what essentially was a cash grab by the University of Florida and Florida State University. That wasn't even the worst of it. The schools just didn't want the University of Miami Medical School to get it.

It was a devastating blow. My father was worn out. He was also angry. Promises had been made to the research staff. Funding demands were growing. No amount of work, not even alongside a legendary Speaker of the House, could blunt the inside dealing.

The fact that it was a Florida senator who denied the award, and steered the funds elsewhere was stunning.

* * *

DAD: I had a lot of friends in politics because I went to Washington, D.C., just about every week in the 1980s. I was very friendly with the Speaker of the House, Tip O'Neill. He was from Boston where I played for seven years with the Patriots. I used to see him at Jimmy's Harborside Restaurant in Boston. He was just a great friend, really terrific.

I knew that if we were going to take the The Miami Project to the next level, then we needed a substantial research grant. Tip took me by the hand and led me to the different committees. That helped a great deal. He knew I had to get the approval of five House committees before we could get any money. I went to Appropriations, Ways and Means—all of them. The Miami Project was a good cause. I didn't have to explain much because they knew all about what we were trying to accomplish.

I was still doing *Inside the NFL* on HBO, so my entrée was smoothed by the fact that most of the staff members were football fans too. We hired a lobbyist in Washington, and she helped us navigate the committees. We were coming down to the end of the congressional session. The RFP was designed and written in such a way that The Miami Project would be the only entity to qualify. I carried this through for nearly a year from start to finish. Everyone knew it was my project.

So what happened? We come right down to the end and suddenly there's competition. The guy who was supposed to shepherd this through was our then-Senator, Bob Graham. He was the one who was supposed to protect us. Instead, the University of Florida and Florida State University saw the RFP, and they put together a competitive grant proposal.

All Graham had to do was go to the president of either school and tell them that I had spent a year getting this where it was and that the money was for a research building for The Miami Project. All he had to do was step in and explain the situation, but he didn't do that. UF, in conjunction with FSU put together a joint proposal, which was oriented more for brain injury with some spinal cord application.

In the final days, they were awarded the $18 million grant. But that wasn't the worst part. The worst part is that they never used the grant because they were never able to execute the plan laid out in their proposal.

I was a member of the Public Health Trust at that time. I was sitting in a meeting when the news came down. It was almost like reliving Marc's injury all over again. Obviously, it wasn't as bad as that day, but it was a punch in the gut. Now we had to go back to square one and try to figure out how we were going to find the funding.

That was almost a mortal blow to The Miami Project. To this day, I'll never understand why Senator Bob Graham didn't protect us. Why didn't he tell UF and FSU that it was his bill, even though I did all the groundwork with my friends from Massachusetts, including the Speaker of the House? There were so many of my friends in Washington who stepped in to help that process along.

I have never counted on anyone else. My feeling has always been, and this is where Marc and I are very much alike, that you can never look back. A person can't make progress if they are always looking behind them. The only way to move ahead is to look forward. You can't make progress if you keep thinking about what's already over. Opportunity is in front of you.

I grew up in a loving family with aunts, uncles, cousins, and grand-parents living right next to us. Everyone was always positive even when it wasn't easy. I started working on a tobacco farm at eleven years of age. I never depended on anybody because I knew what it looked like to take care of yourself and your family. Not that I don't depend on people to perform certain tasks, but I'm not personally dependent upon them. It has certainly been a hallmark of my philosophy, if you want to call it that.

I'm a very stubborn guy. Marc is very stubborn too. It doesn't matter whether Marc is sitting in a wheelchair or not. If Marc wants to do some-thing, then he's going to do it.

So we figured out how to get the money on our own. That's when we established The Buoniconti Fund Board of Directors, a "Who's Who" from the business, sporting, and celebrity worlds.

Instead of raising $18 million, we raised $25 million. We built the building and created the world's leading spinal cord research center.

Chapter 52

"Get Up, Stand Up"

The Miami Project had grown to fifty people spread across multiple buildings when the Washington deal disappeared.

In 1994 we initiated a capital-raising program to find the necessary funds. It was familiar territory for my dad. Rather than rely on people and processes over which we had no control, the decision was made to raise all the money we needed privately.

Gloria Estefan agreed to be the capital campaign chairperson. She had a unique perspective on the importance of the work The Miami Project was doing.

During a 1990 concert tour, she was asleep in a bunk on her tour bus as it was headed to Syracuse, New York, from Scranton, Pennsylvania, when it was forced to stop on a highway along with other vehicles due to a jackknifed eighteen-wheeler. Another truck, unaware of the situation, slammed into the back of Gloria's bus, throwing her from the bunk and resulting in broken vertebrae. She was flown to New York City where surgeons stabilized her back and inserted titanium rods to fuse the broken vertebrae. Gloria had a long recovery to regain her mobility.

With Gloria as the chair, we attracted a world-class board of directors for the capital campaign. The board included: Nike founder and then CEO, Phil Knight; Bob Wright, then president of NBC; Don Keough, then president and COO of Coca-Cola; J. Ira Harris, a Chicago investment banker; and Wayne Huizenga, who founded Waste Management, Blockbuster, AutoNation, and who owned 50 percent of the Miami Dolphins until early 2009; Ray Chambers, the noted private equity investor and philanthropist; and Jack Schneider, chairman of the board.

Bill Ryan, Jr. was paralyzed as a young man while swimming in the ocean off Key Biscayne. His father, Bill Ryan, was an executive at *Post-Newsweek*. Mr. Ryan became a tireless advocate for The Miami Project. He solicited Roger King, the founder and CEO of King World Productions. Mr. King's company distributed the *Oprah Winfrey Show*, *Wheel of Fortune*, *Jeopardy*, and many other shows.

Mr. King hosted the "Roger King Invitational," golf tournaments in Las Vegas and Atlantic City. He opened his Rolodex on behalf of The Miami Project, and in addition to personally covering tremendous costs, raised more than $3 million. Mr. Ryan also connected General Norman Schwarzkopf, who commanded the U.S.-led coalition in the 1991 Gulf War, to The Miami Project. The Schwarzkopf Cup, a fundraising trap-shooting contest, became an annual event.

Despite all these efforts the capital campaign still required significant contribution to make the building a reality. The philanthropist Lois Pope, who was inspired by Christopher Reeve, pledged $10 million.

When the opportunity to speak directly to Florida legislators came up, General Schwarzkopf stepped in to deliver the message. Everyone in Tallahassee knew General Schwarzkopf was speaking that day. There wasn't an empty seat in the chamber the day he spoke.

He banged his fist onto the lectern and, in a booming voice, said, "This charity is squeaky clean. This is a great charity run by great people. You people need to do this. I'm not taking 'no' for an answer."

The bill to match Ms. Pope's $10 million was passed unanimously. We ended up raising $20 million more, which allowed us to further endow and equip the building.

Within three years of the disappointing outcome in Washington, DC, we had the official groundbreaking of the Lois Pope LIFE Center. Ms. Pope provided the largest individual gift, $10 million, and the State of Florida agreed to match it, thanks to the rousing speech delivered by General Norman Schwarzkopf at the state house. In the end, great people find one another.

On October 26, 2000, exactly fifteen years to the day of my injury, the 98,000-square-foot, state-of-the-art Lois Pope LIFE Center opened at the University of Miami Miller School of Medicine. Tom Brokaw flew into South Florida to preside over the ceremony. Gloria Estefan spoke, as did Christopher Reeve, my dad, and me.

In five years we went from an idea to an operational building that was completely funded. It wouldn't have been possible without the extraordinary leadership and tireless work of my father and enough other people to fill a separate book. Among them are Suzie Sayfie, executive director of The Miami Project; her daughter Stephanie Sayfie Aagaard; and the staff's ongoing fundraising efforts.

The impossible is now within sight.

Chapter 53

Back in Black

For the most part, the person injured on the football field is the person who emerged from the hospital. I still enjoyed smoking marijuana and the fact that I was in a chair, at least early on, never dampened my enthusiasm for partying with my friends. I was still a young man. I enjoyed myself.

When I moved out into my own place, life was good. I had been volunteering at The Miami Project for years. I was also living it up and having fun. I was barely thirty years old, single, and relatively healthy, all things considered.

Then I caught a cold during Thanksgiving weekend in 1998. By the following Monday or Tuesday, I was coughing up a lot of phlegm. That really didn't bother me though. It was a minor inconvenience. I don't know why I did this, but I found an old inhaler. It had been prescribed for me about a year earlier for what I thought was a similar cold. I used the inhaler and didn't think much about it. I also took a decongestant. To this day, I really don't know what happened. I think the combination of the inhaler and the decongestant opened up my lungs even more, and that wouldn't have been so bad, but I also smoked. My lungs must have been unusually open, and I sucked smoke and phlegm into my lungs beyond what would have been otherwise possible.

The worst part is that the decongestant dried up the phlegm, which meant it became cemented in my lungs. Suddenly, I couldn't cough. I felt like something was stuck inside my lungs. It actually burned, or destroyed the lining in my bronchial tubes. The process is called atelectasis. It's never gone away.

I kept telling the doctors there was something wrong. I was never short of breath, but I kept feeling something inside me. I went back and forth to the doctor. By December I was on breathing treatments and trying to cough it out. I had a couple of bronchoscopies, which alone are nasty enough. The process involves a tube being inserted through the nose, down into the lungs. My bronchial tubes were bright red, but the doctors didn't see anything in there. I had that done three times. No one ever figured it out. I started doing my own research and talking to my own pulmonary doctors. Finally, I called National Jewish Health in Denver, Colorado. I ended up spending a week there, just my nurse and me.

But there is no such thing as an "ordinary trip" for me. I never take a flight that requires a change of planes. Every time my chair leaves me and is taken by baggage handlers to be stored, there's an excellent chance it's going to come back broken. That's a serious problem. Many times I've reached a destination and had my chair retrieved only to find it in pieces, or missing pieces, and otherwise inoperable.

The process starts at the curb before I ever enter an airport. I have to be dropped off with my nurse, usually from my own van. I drive my chair through the airport to the plane. When I go through security I'm in the chair. Once I get to the plane door, my nurse gets me under the arms and somebody else grabs me under the knees to pick me up. Somebody else has to take the cushion from my chair and put it on my seat. I have no trunk control, so I have to be strapped in securely once I get into the seat.

I book flights in first class because I don't fit in coach. I also have to sit in the very first row, which has the most available room. That's just to get on the plane. My chair has to be reclined flat so it fits in the belly of the plane. I've had airlines tell me they wouldn't take my chair. One airline refused to allow my chair to be stored in the plane because they said the batteries were unsafe. "We're not saying you can't fly, but your chair can't." I had to reverse the entire process and get off the plane. What was I going to do once I landed if I didn't have my chair? When we land I wait for everyone to get off the plane while my chair is brought to the door. The airline has to have an elevator to bring the chair up to the door because it's too heavy and cumbersome to be carried up stairs.

Needless to say, airplane bathrooms are not accessible at all. When I fly to Europe or from coast to coast in the United States, I have to catheterize. That means a blanket has to be held up around me, while my nurse inserts the catheter and drains my bladder.

I have to call in advance to rent a wheelchair-accessible vehicle, which is convenient because I have my nurse along to drive. Then I have to make sure I book the right hotel with the right amenities. The room has to have a roll-in shower because I shower in a special waterproof chair that travels with me as well. I also have to make sure I have connecting rooms so my nurse is easily accessible to me in case I need him.

Hopefully neither I, nor my chair, is damaged along the way. The chair costs $25,000 to $27,000, so it is a big deal if it is damaged. It takes a lot of planning, particularly if I travel somewhere like the Bahamas or Europe, where you can't always count on the amenities. But it can be done.

By the time I arrived in Colorado in February of 1999, my lungs were really causing me problems. My doctor back in Miami kept telling me he couldn't find anything stuck, or otherwise constricting my breathing.

"It is what it is," said one of my doctors.

What kind of answer is that? The doctors in Colorado couldn't find an obstruction, either, but I was heavily congested. What they did find, however, was mold in my lungs. They put me on antifungal medicine. The last day I was in Colorado I received a call that my Nana, my mom's mother, had fallen and hit her head. She was in critical condition with a brain hemorrhage. I quickly returned, and she died two days later on February 27.

That period was the most difficult time in my life post-injury. Not only didn't I know what was happening to my lungs, but there was also an acute psychological element to the entire experience. I couldn't help but think back to the darkest moments. The immediate sensation was a desperate sense of gasping for breath. But this time it was different. I blamed myself for undermining all of the previous efforts. The sense of guilt combined with a creeping hopelessness weighed on me emotionally. I just couldn't believe that despite all the fighting and all the suffering I had basically self-inflicted a wound that might now kill me.

If the idea of contributing to my own demise wasn't enough, my grandmother died, and my parents were divorced. For nearly a year I had a really hard time psychologically. I was confronted by my mortality yet again, only now in a way that came with shame and guilt. For the first time, I really didn't think I was going to survive. I thought the lung problem was going to kill me. What made it all worse, and added to my misery, is that I was so disappointed in myself.

I had worked so hard to get off the respirator. Now I had destroyed my lungs. I felt stupid. The problems became so acute that I had to go back into the hospital and return to the rotating bed to see if that would help. All it did was give me nightmares so disturbing that I had to leave after two days. I wasn't getting any better, and there wasn't any diagnosis.

I could feel myself fading back into the darkness. Only this time I couldn't see any way out.

* * *

NICK JR: I thought Marc was going to die. So did he.

We were talking on the phone one day and he said, "I think I'm going down, brother."

Any sickness with Marc is serious. When they rush Marc back to the University of Miami/Jackson Memorial Hospital, it's serious. He's been in and out of the hospital dozens of times. This time, though, he couldn't breathe properly, and he became very depressed.

I'm not much of a worrier. I said, "Marc, don't overreact. Don't let this get you down. You've made it all the way to this point."

Marc gets very down when he's sick. I can hear it in his voice. He just becomes a different man because sickness has such a compounding effect on him compared to the rest of us. Sickness of any kind drastically affects his body. Then it affects his mood. It probably reminds him of how fragile he is.

There were some depressions that lasted months at a time, but when he came through that episode, I saw Marc have a spiritual change. He blossomed in a way that he hadn't to that point. He grew up.

I don't think Marc has ever been afraid of death. But he became a lot more introspective. He became a lot more caring. Marc was all about Marc before the injury. Now he's willing to help anyone at any time. It was a noticeable change.

Chapter 54

Seeing the Light

I tried everything to find out what was happening inside my lungs. I had an elaborate and large saltwater fish tank in my condominium. I thought maybe there were toxins being released into the air from it, so I had the tank removed. I had people come in and check the air quality. I wanted to give them every opportunity to find something in my environment that was causing me so much discomfort. I even left my place for a few days and checked into a Marriott Hotel on Biscayne Bay, which just happened to be across the street from a small church.

When nothing was found, I was lost. I had reached a crossroads. One day I wheeled myself across the street and into the church. I was out of options. No one had an answer, and I was struggling emotionally as much as physically. I didn't know what was happening to me, or what to do about it. Going into a church was not something I did ordinarily. I was fundamentally disconnected from the entire enterprise of organized religion since grade school.

I had a hard time buying the story of the Catholic Church. I saw nuns use religion as an instrument of control, to scare and modify children's behavior. I saw massive amounts of money spent on self-congratulatory churches. I saw nuns behave badly. I saw priests behave badly. And these actions were directed at children. It was always hard to imagine the benevolent God they preached about in a world filled with pain and suffering. As I grew older, I questioned the most basic philosophical tenets of faith and the existence of any God.

I consider myself a scientist. I form conclusions based on empirical evidence. The more I read, the more I question a story. Whenever it came to my injury, I never thought to inject religion or God into an event that I believed had nothing to do with either. It's the same argument about whether what happens to us in life is free will, fate, destiny, or driven in part by some form of divine intervention. In the end, the debate for me was always irrelevant. Everyone tells me that my injury happened for a reason. My answer has been and always will be that it happened and we created a reason.

In short, the Marc Buoniconti philosophy can be reduced to a simple phrase: Shit happens. It's how you deal with the mess that matters. Regardless of anyone's religious beliefs, nothing changes the fact that each of us is challenged in a variety of ways throughout our lives, whether physically, emotionally, financially, or otherwise. The quality of our lives is determined by the choices we make in response to those challenges. I have always felt that my life was going to be determined by my own actions, one way or the other.

When I decided to head into the church, I wasn't searching for salvation. On the contrary, it was a sign of desperation. I put the question to God almost in the form of an ultimatum:

"OK, so you really exist? Show me. Give me a sign. Prove it."

I recognize the counterargument to this position. I wasn't owed anything from God or anyone else. Yes, it is about faith. But I always had faith in myself. So in a sense I guess it was a crisis of faith. I found ways to overcome whatever problems life presented. This time, I felt my life slipping away.

I didn't hear a crack of lightning or the sound of thunder. When I left that church I figured, "Well, it's up to me once again." For the first time in my life, though, I wasn't sure I had the energy to rise up.

It took me six to eight months before I regained the sense that my life would go on. I've always said that I should have died on the football field. In fact, as much as I've come to understand the human body and its related science, I really don't understand why I *didn't* die on the field. Until the lung problem, I considered everything that came after the initial injury bonus time.

It's not like my life changed all at once the moment I emerged from that church. At the margins, though, I was different. The experience humbled me. It took me back to the ventilator, the rotating bed, and that deep sense of darkness when taking a breath was all I could think about. To some degree, the lung problems made me live parts of that nightmare all over again.

I confronted my mortality. I confronted the notion that life is a precious gift, and that I was in a unique position, as long as I was alive, to impact people's lives positively. I recognized, maybe for the first time, that not everyone had the opportunities I had in front of me. I consciously made the decision that, if I was going to die, then I was first going to accomplish something extraordinary and meaningful not only for me, but for others. It also would serve to wipe the slate clean of past transgressions. I began going out of my way to do what I could to help others; the more extreme the effort, the better.

I knew there were actions that I needed to make amends for, relationships that needed to be fixed. I felt the urge to thank people and let them know that I loved them. It was a matter of readjusting the karma. Years earlier I had borrowed fishing equipment from a friend. One day, I went out and bought him all new equipment. I had it loaded into my van, then drove over to his house. I said, "Here you go, man. Here's everything I borrowed."

I thought, when I'm dead I don't want some guy out there to be able to say, "Marc Buoniconti never returned my fishing gear."

I had another friend who was going through a tough stretch at the same time. I invited him to come live with me for as long as he needed. Then another friend needed a place to stay, so I invited him in too. For a while it was like a halfway house, but that was the way it needed to be.

I quit smoking and drinking. I recognized the changes as they occurred. It was a transformation that I allowed to happen. It was just another in a long line of transformations for me, though. I transitioned from athlete to a person unable to breathe for himself. Then

I transitioned from the ventilator to college graduate. By 1999, I was transitioning toward a completely new chapter.

When no one could tell me what was wrong with my lungs, I tried to find the answer myself. I launched the Bronchitis Center at the University of Miami Miller School of Medicine with a $150,000 grant. Since 2000, we've raised more than $1 million. We have a dozen scientists studying bronchitis and asthma-related problems. I started a wine and cheese festival in Coral Gables with the proceeds going to the American Lung Association. We raised more than $150,000 a year with that event alone.

The work gave me purpose. There was nowhere left to go to find an answer. I looked for one inside myself. I recognized the fact that I had chronic bronchitis. I didn't want anyone else to suffer the way I did.

I saw the light.

I heard the call.

But I emerged shaken and stirred too.

The average person doesn't think twice about the act of taking a breath. For more than eight months that's all I thought about—again. The images that floated into and out of my mind might as well have been the trailer for my own personal horror movie. Imagine reliving your worst nightmare on a reel that keeps playing over and over. Then the clouds slowly began to part. I realized I had squeaked through once more. But this one left a mark. The experience renewed my spirit and refueled my commitment. If I was going to help myself, then I had to do whatever I could to find a cure. I wasn't getting any younger. To say that it had been a tough year is an understatement. I wouldn't have chosen the experience, but I know now that I needed to revisit my personal demons one last time.

That step back into the darkness prepared me to walk out into the light. It was just like a particularly hard hit on the football field. Nothing more. So get up and move on.

* * *

DAD: Marc's lifestyle wasn't conducive to a healthy result. He was doing things he shouldn't have been doing. He was paying the price. I'm not saying that if I were in a wheelchair I wouldn't have been doing some of the things Marc was doing, but the only thing I know is that when your tidal volume is 50 percent of a normal, healthy person, you can't shorten that wick any more. Marc was really, really concerned about his lungs.

That was the biggest slap in the face he could have received. He was never a choirboy. He always took it as far as he possibly could push it. I think he almost pushed himself into the grave.

He finally recognized the fact that if he wanted to be the face of The Miami Project, there was no way he could continue that lifestyle.

It was like turning the *Titanic*.

Graduating from the University of Miami was monumental. It was incredible that he was able to earn his degree given what he had to go through.

After my divorce from Terry, I remarried. One day my wife Lynn told me, and it was so true, "Nick, you can't keep treating Marc as a little boy. He's grown up. He's his own person. He's the one who has to take control of The Miami Project and become its face. You have to let him grow."

The more I heard him speak at the dinners in New York, the more I saw the way he spoke to different people and groups, then seeing him going into The Miami Project on a daily basis and becoming active on the fundraising side, the more I knew my wife was right. Marc was his own man, and he had grown in a lot of different ways.

Marc has a very strong personality. As I've said, when he makes up his mind he's going to do something, there's no turning the clock back. He's going forward.

Nicky and Gina have said that, if an injury like Marc's had to happen to anyone, it happened to the right person in the family. He was the only one who could have handled it the way he has.

Chapter 55

A Call from the Hall

My dad played professional football in an era when an unusual number of the greatest linebackers in history were all playing at the same time. Even though he was the name and face of Miami's legendary "No Name Defense," it took a long time before the Pro Football Hall of Fame came calling.

The phone finally rang early in 2001. We found out the day after the Super Bowl that my father was a finalist. Confirmation came in February during the week of the Pro Bowl in Hawaii. My brother and I were on the phone listening when the league listed the players who would be in the Hall of Fame Class of 2001.

A few years earlier, my dad had pulled me aside.

"If I ever get inducted into the Hall of Fame, I want you to introduce me." The first thing my father said to me after the official announcement was: "Get ready, Marc."

As honored as I was that my dad chose me to introduce him, I also felt a little strange for my brother. Nicky is the oldest. And after all, he is named after our father. If it ever bothered him, he never even hinted that it did. On the contrary, he remained nothing but supportive and encouraging as the day approached.

I spent six months writing the words of that speech. I probably changed it a hundred times. I'd do a little here, a little there. It was one of the proudest moments of my life and it had nothing to do with me.

The opportunity to get up to the podium and talk about my dad, not just the football player but the man and father he is, was an incredible experience. The speech wasn't bad either. It was selected as one of the outstanding speeches in the history of the Hall of Fame.

Is this great or what? Dad, a few years ago, you said, "Marc, if I ever get elected to the Hall of Fame, I want you to introduce me." Well, here we are. And here I am, one lucky person. A kid who grew up with a hero as a dad. And a son who has been asked to introduce his father on the day of his highest honor. I'm humbled by the responsibility of saying so much for so many in so little time . . .

Dad, you've had labels and clichés attached to you throughout your life. Too small. Not NFL material. Overachiever. A quote "intelligent" player. A no-name. But make no mistake about it, you're here today because of what you did on the field. It may have taken the sportswriters twenty years to come around, but now the world knows what your teammates and opponents knew all along. That you were just one great football player.

You once told me, "I never really thought of myself as undersized." Weren't you listening to what people were saying? Maybe you were just too focused to pay attention to those things . . . Your Hall of Fame coach Don Shula had this to say about you, "Without a doubt the key to our great defense in back-to-back Super Bowl seasons was the leadership of our defensive captain, Nick Buoniconti. His tenacity and attention to detail made it happen. He made sure that our "No-Name Defense" was a "no-mistake defense"...

As we know, voters to the Hall of Fame do not consider off-the-field accomplishments. But if they had, they would have found that you have world-class achievements in many areas other than football. In your first few years with the Patriots, you attended Suffolk Law School at night while practicing football in the day. Before you were a Miami Dolphin, you were already a practicing attorney in the off-season.

But just as remarkable as your achievements on the field and in the boardroom is your unselfish dedication to making a difference in the lives of others. And Dad, this is probably where you excel above all else.

This great game of football has given our family its brightest moments and its darkest days. Dad, 85 was your lucky number. But 1985 brought some rough times for the Buoniconti family. Early that year, you lost your own dad to cancer, and then in October, I had my paralyzing injury playing linebacker for The Citadel. Looking into your eyes, I saw a mask of pain and fear transform into that familiar look of determination. I knew you were getting ready for our biggest challenge. So, when they started using labels for me and telling you all the medical clichés that I'd never walk again, that I'd need a machine to breathe for me, that paralysis can't be cured, once again you didn't listen. You made a bedside promise to do everything and anything to help me walk again. Your promise that October day 16 years ago became The Miami Project to Cure Paralysis, the world's largest, most comprehensive spinal cord research center. It is a symbol of hope for hundreds of thousands of Americans who are awaiting a cure.

Dad, you never believed the labels and limitations others ascribed to you. Instead you faced each challenge head-on and made believers out of them. So in closing, I've got a label for you that I've never heard mentioned. Dad, as I look at all the things they say you couldn't do, it seems to me that you're just not a very good listener.

Who would have thought that the son of an Italian baker from the south end of Springfield, Massachusetts, would go on to run a Fortune 500 company? Or that a guy with a degree in economics would be helping to make medical history? Or that a 13th-round pick of the fledgling AFL would today be inducted into the Pro Football Hall of Fame?

Dad, you've always been by my side and have been more of a father to me than I could have ever imagined. The best father one could hope for. Whatever it is you got inside you, we see it, we feel it, and it gives each of us a little more reason to believe.

It was one of the most unbelievable weekends of my life. I remember thinking, "My life has already been unbelievable. Sometimes I can't believe it myself."

* * *

NICK JR: My father has earned everything he's ever gotten through grit and determination. It's that old-fashioned kind of work ethic that he grew up seeing in the men and women of his family.

I'm not sure the Buonicontis are thought of as a philosophical family. We're just doers. We get up in the morning and do what needs to be done. It's not a whole lot more complicated than that.

My dad set a goal and achieved it—the right way, first class every time. I've seen him tired but I've never heard him complain. My dad has never failed at anything. He's been a success every place he's gone, whether it was football or business.

When my dad chose Marc to introduce him at the Hall of Fame, it never occurred to me to be jealous. After all that Marc has done, I would have chosen him too. I was just proud to be a Buoniconti.

Chapter 56

Ring Ceremony

The effects of a catastrophic injury extend outward like the ripples of a wave. For some, the experience of being involved, even at a distance can be life-altering to a degree that is hard to fathom.

By 2005, I had been in a wheelchair longer than I had been out of one. As the twentieth anniversary of my injury approached, I received a call from a former teammate and friend, Joel Thompson. Joel was on the field that day, a linebacker just like me. As the play developed, Joel dove at the ball carrier, Herman Jacobs, and tripped him up, beginning the sequence of events that changed my life.

Joel and I had talked only once after the injury. When he called, the initial conversation was about how badly he felt because so much time had passed between us. He wanted to do whatever he could to re-establish our friendship and make up for lost time. That included his commitment to launch a Buoniconti Fund chapter in Atlanta where he lived. He decided to come down to Miami for just a weekend. Real friends seem to have the ability to remain connected over long periods of time and distance, even without direct contact. It never occurred to me that Joel wasn't my friend or that our relationship had changed. We just needed to catch up.

When Joel arrived, we picked up more or less where we had left off. We spent very little time talking about The Citadel, though. That is, until he came into my bedroom. The closet door was open.

"Take a look," I said.

Inside were my two garrison caps, along with the "shako"—an ornamental plume—used for marching. My jersey was hanging there too. Everything was neatly and perfectly positioned. The Citadel might have forgotten me, but I never forgot The Citadel.

Later that afternoon, Joel asked if I had thought about making amends with the school.

"No. Not really. I've never thought it would happen."

For the most part, that was the truth.

"Well, what do you think about going back and trying to iron it all out? Would you be open to burying the hatchet?"

"Joel, I wouldn't mind having that conversation. There's one condition, though. I'm not going to reach out to them. They have to reach out to me. I'm not going to make the first move."

He paused, and with a look of humility said: "Marc, I'm sorry. I'm just sorry I haven't talked to you all this time. I didn't know how to talk to you. I didn't know what to say or how to say it. It ends right now. I'll make it up to you, man. I want to try to do this for you. Where do I start?"

"Joel, I never took it personally. I understand. But if you are going to approach The Citadel, then you have to start at the top. Call the president of the school."

That's the way it was left. Joel headed back to Atlanta. I went back to work on Monday. It was a nice idea. Although time hadn't healed all wounds, it had softened the edges. Both sides needed a sense of closure. What followed was beyond my imagination.

Behind the scenes and unknown to me, another one of our teammates, John Stephens, worked with Joel to pry the gates open and reconnect me and The Citadel. Joel not only spoke to the then interim-president, General Roger Clifton Poole, but he traveled from Atlanta to Charleston on numerous occasions to make sure his thoughts and sentiments were articulated in person. He spoke to the president and other leaders within the school administration, including Billy

Jenkinson, the Chairman of the Board of Visitors, which operated as the school's Board of Directors. Meanwhile, John worked the political levers locally in Charleston.

A few months later, the first official invitation arrived. I was invited to Corps Day, the official celebration that takes place every March. They made the first move. They had finally reached out.

I shared the news immediately with my family. I can't recall exactly with whom I spoke first, but it was important for me to hear everyone's take. My mom, Gina, and Nicky all felt positive about the development, and thought it was a great opportunity to heal old wounds and mend broken hearts. My father, on the other hand, is the one who has always been a bit more reserved about the notion of forgiving and forgetting. He responded with indifference and skepticism. There was a part of me that agreed with him. There's nothing simple about burying two decades of frustration and heartache. I'd be returning to the scene of the crime, so to speak, for the first time since the lawsuit.

Sometimes too much pride can be a detriment to progress. Had this invitation occurred ten years earlier, I don't think I would have had the will or maturity to appreciate the greater good. I'm pretty sure this was a reflection of the "new" Marc since my medically induced spiritual epiphanies.

I accepted the invitation. We made the drive up to Charleston from Miami in my van, along with Lance, my nurse, and my friend Fatty McConnon. Lt. General John W. Rosa had replaced General Poole as president. Colonel Dick and others were in the room when I arrived for the meeting. Billy Jenkinson said the first words:

"Welcome home!"

I felt an immediate emotional release. After a long and trying twenty years, I really felt like I was home again. Contrary to previous trips back—the trial, my classmates' graduation—I was being welcomed with open arms by The Citadel and its administration. The meeting was also about retiring my jersey. The schedule was set. My jersey would be retired in a ceremony during halftime of The Citadel-Elon game that fall. What I still didn't know was all that my friends did and would continue to do behind the scenes to make this happen.

My father was reluctant to attend the jersey ceremony, but he agreed at the last minute. I understood my dad's reluctance. To put the past behind and embrace the source of so much pain is a difficult pill to swallow for someone as principled as my dad. Even before I agreed to go back and make amends, he and I had several conversations. In the end, he recognized that going back to The Citadel was just another opportunity to turn a negative situation into a positive experience.

My family and a handful of my closest friends made the trip to Charleston. The weekend's festivities started with a gathering in the courtyard of the Alumni House. As I approached the courtyard I noticed the group was larger than I expected. Once we were settled, John stood up to make a short speech. I had no idea what was coming.

When John finished talking, he pulled out a Citadel ring, walked over to me, and placed it on my finger. I was overwhelmed. I broke down and started crying. Through the tears, I looked out and saw my teammates and another group of my classmates from F-Troop in the courtyard. All of them had come together on my behalf. They never said a word about all the efforts they had made. Then I looked up, and a group of Air Force fighter jets, organized by Lt. General Rosa, executed a flyover in my honor. It was all emotionally overwhelming.

The ring signifies more than just graduating from The Citadel. It represents a cadet's symbolic connection to the school. Until that day, no ring had ever been awarded to anyone, under any circumstances, who had failed to graduate from The Citadel. Not even in the 1960s at the height of the Vietnam War, when kids were being killed, or permanently disabled and unable to finish school, did anyone receive a ring without first receiving a diploma. The administration remained resolute even when doing so appeared to be unconscionable.

I didn't find out until later that Joel and John, along with dozens of my classmates and teammates, had been unrelenting in their lobbying for the ring. John made multiple trips to the campus. He made presentations to various members of the school's hierarchy. Once, when John found out the Board of Visitors had scheduled a vote on the matter and that no one would be there to speak on my behalf, he made sure he was there in person and demanded to be heard in the meeting.

After months and months of work, countless hours spent fighting red tape, and tracking down classmates, John presented a petition to the Board of Visitors signed by all my classmates. My friends acted exactly as we had been trained to act. When a fellow soldier was down, step up. They acted with passion, resolve, selflessness, and most of all, honor. The school might have been prepared to move on and let others debate whether it had left one of their own on the battlefield. Not my friends. Colonel Dick and a few others were so impressed with the efforts made by John, Joel, and the others that they voted unanimously to give me a ring.

The next day my jersey was retired at halftime. We won the game and the team presented me with the game ball. It took twenty years for us to overcome the impact of a single moment. And within twenty-four hours, it was all behind me. Before it happened, I wasn't sure reconciliation was even possible after so much time had passed. I spoke to my father about it. He never wavered on his stance. His was a selfless act of supporting his son, just as he had done my entire life. He wasn't anxious to extend an olive branch, much less rewrite history. But he was willing to do it for me.

The weekend confirmed something that I was never entirely sure about. I knew that I had made the right decision. I realized and appreciated the efforts of John, Joel, and others to clean the slate. People such as Colonel Dick, Billy Jenkinson, and President Rosa weren't obligated to do anything. Their legacy would have remained intact whether they lifted a finger on my behalf or not.

To have my family, all of them, as well as my childhood friends, at The Citadel for the first time in twenty years provided a great sense of closure on terms more positive and inspiring than I could have imagined.

Chapter 57

Delayed Impact

As the weekend at The Citadel wound down, the conversation turned to all the people who should have been there but weren't. Somebody brought up the names of players on other teams that we played that season. Joel mentioned Herman Jacobs, the guy carrying the ball for East Tennessee State when our lives collided in Johnson City.

"He should be here," Joel said.

It wasn't like anyone actually knew Herman, or where he lived. Just the fact he had been involved in the play was enough. I looked at Joel.

"Would you try to find him? Herman should be here next year when we all get together again."

It took six or seven months to locate him.

Then I got the call from Joel. "Marc, I found Herman. Here's his phone number. Give him a call. He's looking forward to talking to you."

I took the number and gave Herman a call. We spoke for ten or fifteen minutes. We talked around the edges of life—small talk—nothing too personal or intimate. But I told him it would be great to have him at The Citadel for next year's reunion.

A couple weeks later Joel called back.

"So, did you talk to Herman?"

"Yeah, we spoke."

"Well?"

"It was fine. We just talked for a few minutes."

"That's it?"

Joel couldn't believe that Herman and I didn't have an immediate emotional connection on the telephone. What I didn't know is that in the months that followed, Joel spoke to Herman a few more times. It wasn't until the next reunion rolled around that I came to know the degree to which my injury had affected Herman.

When I went back to The Citadel to have my jersey retired, I heard dozens of stories from people who had been affected by my injury. It was disorienting at first. A number of my teammates, friends, class-mates, and people from the school never forgot what happened that day. It affected each of them differently. Until that first reunion I rarely talked to anyone from The Citadel about the injury. The more we talked, the more I found out what a significant impact my injury had on so many people. I guess I didn't appreciate what they had to go through on campus, especially with the lawsuit and the negative feelings it engendered. So when Herman and I met in person, I was better prepared mentally and emotionally for his story in a way that I wouldn't have been a year earlier.

Herman is a gentle giant of a man with thick, powerful legs and an equally strong, compact body. But other than an abiding passion for football, our stories couldn't be more different. Herman is Afri-can-American, soft-spoken, and tremendously humble. When I was growing up running around the Orange Bowl on Saturday afternoons with an All-Pro linebacker for a father, Herman was navigating Tam-pa's toughest neighborhoods in a home broken by violence and harsh economics. I could see my father play professional football on televi-sion every Sunday. Herman was five years old when he watched his father get gunned down in broad daylight in the small front yard of his house. My brother went to Duke on a football scholarship and became a lawyer. Herman's older brother ended up being shot to death in drug-related mayhem only weeks before he was scheduled to move in with Herman in Johnson City.

I couldn't have known that Herman's anguish had so many roots. When he was in middle school, he played defense. One day he raced across the line of scrimmage, no doubt moving through and around players trying to block him. He slammed into a slender quarterback on the opposing team. When Herman pushed himself off the turf, the kid didn't move. Herman's hit temporarily paralyzed Henry Mull. Herman never played defense again, which is why he was a running back on that Saturday when our lives collided on the field.

I didn't know any of this when Herman and I first spoke in Charleston in 2006. I hadn't seen him since the trial. He was a witness for the defense. The longer we talked, the more I realized that our collision had created another deep and emotional trauma for him. It was as if his unique history—rough childhood, previous experience with a spinal cord injury, and sense of guilt about my injury—broke to the surface in a rush he couldn't control. All these years Herman had been pulled under. He couldn't break free from the demons long enough to save himself.

In a sense, I wasn't the only one dying on the field that day.

Herman was like a dormant volcano ready to explode when Joel found him. He had kept so much emotion bottled up over his guilt about my injury that his life literally crumbled around him. We brought Herman into the fold at a critical time in his life. He was working in a small restaurant in Johnson City just outside the shadow of the football stadium where our lives intersected.

He had become a recluse, drawn deeply into himself under the weight of all the emotions leading up to and including our fateful meeting. He was living life day to day with no passion, purpose, direction, or goals. He was just passing through a life he wouldn't have wished on anyone. I could see that his entire situation was depressing. I could see that he was in a deep hole and drowning. He needed to get out of Johnson City. He needed to leave the scene of the crime and find a way out from under the cloud that had enveloped him. I had a simple question for him:

"What are your dreams?"

He had a simple answer.

"I always wanted to be a chef."

Chapter 58

Internal Paralysis

HERMAN: There were three linebackers I'll never forget. But none of them hit as hard as Marc did.

I knew Marc was hurt badly when we collided. That's about all I remember of the game. Other than Marc lying on the field and emergency personnel rushing to his side, I don't remember a thing. I didn't even find out who won the game until the next day.

In the moments after Marc's injury, I pretty much, right then and there, gave up the game of football. It was the second time something like that had happened in my life. I couldn't understand why. To me, the game wasn't about hurting people. It was fun. It was a way to release anger and frustration that built up over the days and weeks. Football was an outlet for me. I could get out onto the field and be myself. When the game devolved into a life or death situation, I didn't want any part of it.

I was standing on the sidelines as the doctors ran out onto the field and attended to Marc. I heard comments that suggested he might be paralyzed. I knelt down on one knee, took my helmet off and shook my head in disbelief. In the days and years that followed I must have been told the same thing a thousand times:

"Herman, it's just a game. It's not your fault."

I understood how others could say it wasn't my fault. But people mean a lot more to me than the game ever did. I knew you could play football and maybe one day make a lot of money. My two biggest idols, the people I looked up to and studied, were Walter Payton and Earl Campbell. I watched those guys. I read books about them. I studied their styles and paid attention to how hard they trained; when I went out onto the field that's who I tried to portray. Off the field, I tried to emulate the way they carried themselves. I knew Walter Payton was famous for how hard he worked in the offseason. I followed his example. I was working hard too.

On the day we played The Citadel, scouts for the San Francisco 49ers, the Chicago Bears, and quite a few other NFL teams were there to watch me play. But football lost all its meaning the moment Marc was hurt. I understood what those scouts meant to my future. But it was over.

I finished out the season, though I can't recall anything beyond that game. It's a lot like my father dying. I don't remember much about the incident. There are a few moments between seeing him come home and getting out of his truck. The next thing I remember is my father being shot and killed. After that the only thing I recall is that we moved, and I started school somewhere else. We didn't move until a year after he was killed. I had to ask my family questions like, where is my father buried? What happened after he was killed? I didn't remember anything.

Around the time of Marc's injury, I found out my brother was selling drugs. That bothered me too. In the neighborhood where we grew up, if you didn't get out, then you got into the drug business. I couldn't tell you the number of kids who got themselves into trouble with drugs, using, selling, or both. My brother turned out to be one of them.

I was always different. I had a lot of friends, but I didn't always like what they did. I was one of those kids who stood up and let the others know that I didn't want any part of that scene. That's one of the reasons I was able to go to college. I wasn't a good student at first. Then I met friends who were smart and made good grades. They inspired me to do the same.

I wasn't always a calm, collected person. After my father was killed, I became one of those mean individuals. I stayed in trouble for a long time. By the time I reached high school, the anger had washed out of me. Football became my escape. I learned to leave everything I had on the field.

Even in college, I never went out after a game like most of my teammates. I was tired. I didn't have any energy left to do anything except sleep.

When the game ended against The Citadel, I went directly to the hospital to see about Marc. I felt responsible in a way that's hard to describe. I didn't agree with the analysis that it wasn't my fault. I believed that I could have done something differently. The wife of a graduate assistant in my dormitory gave me a ride to the hospital. On the way there, I told her that football was over for me.

Marc wasn't in any condition to see anyone but immediate family. His brother Nicky came out and talked to me. He thanked me for coming. As far as I know, no one else from my team went to the hospital that night. From that day forward, people told me they saw a change in me. I noticed it too. I slipped into a big hole as the days and years went by.

I finished the season, but I only have vague memories of anything that happened following Marc's injury. I do know we went 0-10-1. I don't remember how the games played out. I came back for my senior year even though I didn't want to. It was a roller-coaster season. If I tell somebody I'm going to do something, then I do it. I told the coaches that I would play, so I did. I wasn't afraid, but I no longer had the confidence, the joy, the drive, or love for the game. I don't know whether NFL scouts came around during my senior season because I didn't care one way or another. I couldn't wait for it to be over. The coaches stayed on my back, but I was done.

"We know you can play better. Run the ball harder. Why aren't you doing it?"

They knew I wasn't playing well. They just didn't know why.

I was in junior high school when Henry Mull got hurt. I was playing defense, and I tackled Henry. He became paralyzed for a while. I refused ever to play defense again. I loved defense. I loved playing outside linebacker and free safety. I was out there to have fun, talk trash, and compete. I wasn't there to hurt anybody.

I went to a psychologist at East Tennessee State because life was becoming too much for me to handle. I became deeply depressed in the months and years following Marc's injury.

When I was growing up a friend of mine, Junior Rhodes, took me to church. I started to go with him on a regular basis in ninth grade. I liked church too. I slowly saw myself changing. I liked myself not being angry. I liked myself more than I did when I was making someone mad. Even when Henry got hurt, I stayed with the church. I became president of the Fellowship of Christian Athletes my junior and senior years in high school.

It was difficult to reconcile my faith with what happened to Marc. I have always believed things happen for a reason. But I couldn't figure out the reason for Marc's injury. Did Marc's injury and my brother's death threaten my faith? Yes. Did I stop going to church as much as I did before those things happened? Yes.

I had a lot of questions. The psychologist told me I was going into a depression. Actually, I was scared. He told me to call him anytime of the day or night and I did. He recognized I had a lot of questions and not a lot of answers. He told me I wasn't a bad person, just a person to whom bad things had happened. How do you explain that to a kid who left high school at eighteen, then within four years all this happens, and his nearest relative is more than six hundred miles away?

No one understood. No one had the money to take me back home. My mother was working two jobs. I couldn't tell her how everything was affecting me because she had enough to worry about. I was the only one to graduate from high school in our family. I didn't leave college right away. I kept trying. I just didn't have the drive. I kept working toward my degree, but I had a hard time studying. I had a hard time getting out of bed in the morning. I just didn't want to do anything.

In some ways I was paralyzed too.

Chapter 59

Welcome to My World

Herman was having a hard time. It reminded me of the moment just days after my injury when I couldn't speak because of the tubes inserted in my nose and throat. I looked into my dad's eyes, wanting to say: "Help me, Dad." I couldn't say what I needed to communicate, but he knew.

I could see the same kind of desperation in Herman's eyes. He couldn't say the words either. What I saw in his eyes was: "Help me, Marc." He didn't ask, but I knew that I could help him change his life whether he expected me to or not.

I asked Herman to visit me in Miami. A few months later, he brought his entire family down for a week. I set them up in an apartment in my building. By then I had already made a phone call to the culinary school, Johnson & Wales University, and set up a meeting.

I went to the school, explained Herman's situation to the president, and asked him what they could do for him. I had meetings arranged, as well as job interviews set up for Herman's wife, who had been trained as a nurse. Very quickly I could see Herman was being dragged down as much by his own memories as his reality. His wife was very negative. She had physical problems that made it difficult to walk. It was her attitude that weighed on him. We arranged for her to see some doctors to help her figure out the severity of her infirmities.

By the end of the week, she had a job lined up. The people at Johnson & Wales did everything they could do to make it possible for Herman to be admitted into their program. They provided a scholarship. Along with a Pell Grant, he could attend the school for about $300 per semester. But he had some decisions to make.

I'm sure he was overwhelmed by it all. It's not easy for anybody to pick up their family and move eight hundred miles away. We had a number of phone conversations in the weeks that followed. The more we talked, the more he warmed to the idea of changing his life.

I wanted to make one point crystal clear:

"Herman, don't do this for me. You have no obligation to me. I'm not going to harp on it one way or another. It's an opportunity, but you have to be the one to make the move. Do this for yourself or don't do it at all."

On his own, Herman contacted the school, submitted all the necessary paper work, had his transcripts sent, and did everything else required. He called me a couple weeks before school started. He had been trying to figure out how to get the cost of room and board covered because the financial assistance wasn't enough. Oh well, I thought. It looks like I'm going to have a new roommate for a while.

Herman came back to Miami and moved in with me. As with most things, his presence turned out to be a blessing in disguise. On the morning of December 2, 2008, Lance, my nurse, had a heart attack. When Lance returned to work, he couldn't lift heavy objects for a while. That meant Herman had to handle my daily transfers from the bed to my chair in the morning and back again at night.

It seemed fitting. I needed Herman as much as he needed me. We needed each other.

Two years later, I was like a proud parent when I attended Herman's graduation from Johnson & Wales. He earned an Associate's Degree in Culinary Arts. His mother and sister joined us at the ceremony, followed by a celebratory lunch at Smith & Wollensky's on South Beach.

Herman works for a new restaurant group called PDQ. He is the operations director at one of their franchise stores in Tampa, where he lives. More than thirty years after our lives collided on a football field during an otherwise insignificant game in Johnson City, Tennessee, we have both come full circle.

Since my injury I've dedicated my life to curing paralysis. While I continue to dream of being on my feet once again, for now I take pride in opportunities to involve myself in the lives of those who need hope, a helping hand.

Herman, too, had been paralyzed.

* * *

MOM: Whether it's taking care of his grandparents or interacting with the guy cleaning the street, Marc is incredibly thoughtful. He's so in tune with other people's feelings. He's very much into helping his fellow man, which is why nothing surprised me.

When Herman came back into our lives it was like, "Oh well, set another place at the table."

I remember reading once that when you die, God's not going to ask you how much money you made, or even what you did with the money you made. His only question is going to be: How were you to your fellow man?

The answer to that question either gets you into heaven, or it doesn't. Even if Marc isn't religious in the traditional sense, he's actually more religious than all the rest of us. He's reached a level beyond religion. He doesn't have to go to church. He's already connected. He has the right idea about what we were put here to do—to serve our fellow man. I think people would be surprised by how spiritual he is.

We can't imagine where life will take us if only we're willing to go along for the ride. It's remarkable that I can say this, but it's true. There are so many people in this world who are better off because of Marc's injury.

Chapter 60

The Science

It has been a remarkable journey for me to witness and participate in a scientific revolution in brain and spinal cord injury research. I have always remained hopeful that I would be able to take advantage of the advances in research to improve my quality of life, and gain independence. I hope and pray for the same for the millions of others worldwide in wheelchairs.

Now more than ever, I believe that I have a chance to walk again thanks to the research breakthroughs at The Miami Project.

Early on after my injury, my father, Dr. Barth Green, and other supporters were challenged by the question of deciding in which method our research efforts would be directed. Two schools of thought permeated the discussion. The first was to be a fundraising organization that acted as a middleman between the donor and the research organizations. For example, the parent organization would solicit funds from donors and then request proposals from different research organizations and universities throughout the U.S. and beyond. A scientific review board would vet proposals.

The second option was to establish one center by recruiting a multidisciplinary team of researchers to work together and to utilize the tools of collaboration to improve outcome measures. That model would allow us as directors to have greater oversight and control over decisions and the direction of research.

We felt strongly that if we wanted to recruit the best of the best, we would need to ensure that the researchers were provided the optimal resources as incentive. To that end, it was decided to choose the latter option to be able to have the quality control and centralized leadership to achieve our lofty, but realistic goal of curing paralysis.

By 2016, and under the direction of Dr. W. Dalton Dietrich, our building is now the most advanced research facility for investigating traumatic brain injury including concussions, spinal cord injury, stroke, and other neurological diseases such as Multiple Sclerosis.

What separates The Miami Project from many other research organizations is that we are one of only a few centers in the world that combine expertise in basic, translational, and clinical science with quality of life programs. This comprehensive approach allows us to take advantage of the full spectrum of experts in multiple disciplines. We design research programs from basic science to clinical research with the ultimate goal of initiating new human clinical trials. This strategy has proven to be successful, and has set the stage for the final push toward restoring function and sensation to the paralyzed.

The science would not be possible, however, without the unique contributions of many very special people. One of them is Christine Lynn. The renowned philanthropist donated $10 million to start The Human Clinical Trials Initiative, and then she provided an extraordinary $25 million gift to build The Christine E. Lynn Rehabilitation Center for The Miami Project to Cure Paralysis. I will never be able to thank her enough for her vision and generosity.

She is not alone. Others including Stuart Rahr, Micky and Madeleine Arison; Richard Gray; Mark Dalton; Barbara and Tom Brokaw; Bob Costas; Jack Nicklaus; Gloria and Emilio Estefan; Edie Laquer; Paul and Swanee Di Mare; the Bantle Family; the Chambers Family; all the Great Sports Legends; and the many incredible donors and volunteers who have made the march to stand up inevitable.

Our scientific breakthroughs are remarkable. We have been approved by the Food and Drug Administration (FDA) to conduct human trials with Schwann cells. Schwann cells are found in animals and humans and reside in the peripheral nervous system, which are extremities that branch out from the central nervous system (the brain and spinal cord). Schwann cells are so important because central nervous system cells have an extremely difficult time repairing themselves after injury.

When someone endures a brain or spinal cord injury, it sets off a cascade of traumatic consequences resulting in a hostile environment for cell survival and regeneration. Inflammation is a primary cause of the secondary damage, accompanied by hemorrhaging and the release of potentially neurotoxic chemicals that induce cells to die by several mechanisms in necrosis and programmed cell death or apoptosis. The combination of all these primary and secondary factors makes it extremely difficult for any kind of natural recovery. Due to the circumstances, three main things occur when suffering an injury to the central nervous system:

- The cells in and around the site die;
- The axons, which branch out from each cell and communicate with other cells, are damaged;
- The myelin, a protective barrier that surrounds the cells and axons, which allow for the transmission of signals between cells, gets damaged.

In order to develop more effective treatments, and ultimately to cure paralysis, all three of these problems must be addressed. That is why we are so excited about the future of Schwann cells research. Schwann cells encompass the ability to address many of the issues that we are facing in trying to regenerate the central nervous system. Schwann cells have the ability to regenerate, even after being exposed to trauma. Schwann cells release a natural chemical called nerve growth factors that act as "fertilizer" and improve the regeneration process. Last, they possess the ability to repair and replace the myelin that had been damaged. This process is known as re-myelination. It is the combination of all these factors that encouraged us to begin the process of growing human Schwann cells, studying their behavior in a petri dish, moving to animal studies, and now into human studies.

The process is important because safety is critical. We have to be certain we do no harm. We continued to discover methods that improved the function of Schwann cells. For now, the work involves only Schwann cells rather than additional drugs, genes, molecules, and other chemicals that help the Schwann cells proliferate in the areas around an injury. That is because we need to control the variables.

We received FDA approval to conduct the first human trial on patients with subacute injuries. A subacute injury is one that has just occurred, as opposed to a chronic injury. Since then, we have transplanted Schwann cells into several people with subacute thoracic spinal cord injury. That meant that recruiting subjects wasn't easy. In fact, upon approval the initial subacute patients were people not yet even paralyzed.

There is a very well-defined protocol for the trial that involves a myriad of variables including the type, location, and severity of injury, age of the person, the number of other complications, and other inclusion/exclusion criteria. Our approach uses a person's own Schwann cells to avoid any autoimmune rejection. But a person who has suffered a catastrophic injury, by definition, has a compromised autoimmune system. We have completed our subject enrollment for the subacute trial and are now recruiting subjects for a second chronic human Schwann cell trial again approved by the FDA. For this trial, spinal cord-injured subjects who have had an injury for at least 1 year are included. Also, a greater numbers of Schwann cells will be transplanted and the subjects will undergo an extensive rehabilitation protocol to help promote functional improvements. The trial thus far has resulted no significant risk factors associated with transplanting Schwann cells into individuals with severe spinal cord injury. Is there efficacy? Based on the animal studies, there is reason to believe that there could be benefits also seen in humans.

There are other exciting developments involving stem cell transplants. We work with companies to help develop the best methods of utilizing those cells for regeneration after brain and spinal cord injuries. We are also interested in the potential benefits of combining the stem cells with our Schwann cells. We believe this could increase the potential for more regeneration and sensory and motor recovery. In some studies, the stem cells are transplanted around the lesion site as opposed to injections directly into the lesion cavity. Other stem cell treatments include systemic injections that represent a less invasive approach than cell injections directly into the cord.

All these years of research is not just about impacting the future. We have changed the lives of thousands of people who in earlier days would have had no hope. Our Scientific Director, Dr. Dietrich, has been working for years on neuroprotection for acute and chronic injuries. When a person suffers a catastrophic injury there is a robust inflammatory and free radical response. The goal for neuroprotection is to find a way to decrease damaging secondary mechanisms of injury including inflammatory to protect vulnerable brain regions.

During the initial injury, the primary inflammatory process can create significant damage. However, it's the secondary injury brought on by the inevitable inflammation during the days, hours, and even minutes following the primary injury that is even more significant to control. If doctors can intervene early enough after the primary injury with drugs or induced therapeutic hypothermia (i.e., mild cooling), then you can mitigate the secondary injury brought on by the inflammation. The idea for inducing controlled hypothermia after spinal cord injury is similar to putting an ice pack on a broken ankle. This strategy can be accomplished by cooling the body service with cooling blankets or systemically cooling by injecting ice-cold saline or using intravascular cooling catheters. These strategies are being used and tested in a variety of neurological patient populations including stroke, cardiac arrest, postnatal hypoxic encephalopathy, and brain trauma. The Miami Project with the Department of Neurological Surgery is now testing therapeutic hypothermia after acute cervical spinal cord injuries.

The practice of cooling spinal cord patients early after injury is still not widely used at this time. That's why we are in the process of conducting the first multicenter clinical trial to understand and measure the actual effects on safety and functional outcome. Dr. Dietrich gave a speech at a seminar about using this hypothermia technique. The Buffalo Bills' team physician, Dr. Andrew Cappuccino, happened to be present. A few months later, one of the Bills' players, Kevin Everett, went down on the field suffering a cervical spinal cord injury nearly the exact type as mine. Dr. Cappuccino was one of the first people onto the field. He took it upon himself to induce the hypothermia treatment, which was a controversial decision.

We had been studying the treatment for years and there had been numerous scientific papers written on its success. There are skeptics, of course, and that's understandable. But here's what we know. Six months after his injury, Kevin Everett walked into The Miami Project and shook hands with Dr. Dietrich. We don't have irrefutable "scientific" proof that Dr. Cappuccino's decision in the heat of the moment led to the player's ability to avoid life in a wheelchair. But I'm sure this was evidence enough for Kevin Everett. We believe that the science developed by The Miami Project helped produced Everett's positive results.

Another emerging and exciting area of research at The Miami Project, under the direction of Dr. Gillian Hotz, is preventing and managing the effects of concussion. Prior to the NFL settlement in 2016 to former players for their concussions and traumatic brain injuries caused by playing the game, there have been rule changes and many research studies and clinical trials initiated. All are trying to improve the equipment, sideline concussion evaluations, and treatments as well as increase the education of coaches, athletic trainers, players, and parents at all levels of play. Since 2012, we have implemented a Countywide Concussion Program with 6 steps to safer play protocol for all public and private high school football players as well as for others playing contact sports.

The protocol includes baseline and sideline testing, clinical evaluation, a gradual return to play, and a concussion injury surveillance system. Most recently, Dr. Hotz has been awarded a large grant from Scythian Biosciences to study the Pre-clinical and Clinical Effects of Cannabinoids (CBD) on MTBI. Current research is all pointing to the positive effects of CBD with headaches, pain, anxiety, and so forth.

I've always taken the approach that there's a possibility I'll never get out of this chair. I'm in a chair until proven otherwise. I'm paralyzed until proven otherwise. Some days I'm frustrated by the lack of progress. Then there are days when research comes to light that looks positive. I have cautious optimism. I've always thought that it's simply a matter of time. The question is: Do I have enough time? Am I going to live long enough to see a cure and benefit from it personally? A cure is going to be found. It's going to happen; whether or not it's going to happen in a timeframe that benefits me remains to be seen.

I often feel like I'm being pulled in two different directions. One part of me is chomping at the bit to try almost anything to get out of this chair. On the other hand, I understand the complexity of the science involved. My life is at a point now where I am at least as comfortable waiting on the science rather than taking a chance and compromising my delicate state and quality of life. I have a lot to lose. If my injury were one level up my spine, then I'd be back on the respirator. I have to be very careful. Right now, I'm an observer like everyone else. I'm probably the biggest cheerleader, though.

I challenge anybody to pick any disease. Then start from zero, and in thirty years produce the breakthroughs we have experienced. The Miami Project has changed the global scientific community's attitude toward paralysis research.

I do know this: If I could move my arms and feed myself that would represent a tremendous change in my life. If I could breathe easier, have better bowel and bladder function, then any of those would dramatically improve my quality of life.

It's all about independence. For someone who has experienced such a drastic loss of independence, any incremental reclamation is, relatively speaking, monumental.

* * *

DAD: All of the work will be fulfilling to me when we take the clinical trials to humans and the positive results finally become standard of care. Then, through the research, we will have helped someone who hasn't been able to move his hands is suddenly able to pick up a fork, or scratch his nose.

Until that day comes I'm not resting.

I can't rest because there is so much invested—time, money, research, and energy— by so many people that I want to see them rewarded.

I want to see people like Marc rewarded. It's been a long haul and we've been pushing that rock up the hill for a long time.

Chapter 61

Say "No" to Football

In addition to our primary focus on spinal cord injury research, The Miami Project is now considered one of the leading centers in the world for concussion research.

My interest began more than a decade ago when I had discussions with former New York Giants linebacker and NFL Hall of Famer Harry Carson. Harry was one of the first former players to document the effects to his brain of multiple concussions throughout his NFL career. He helped raise awareness and identify concussion as the cause of his reduced cognitive function.

At the time, I was agnostic. I played football at a high level. I had suffered concussions. We looked at them as part of the game. My discussions with Harry made me think about the short- and long-term effects. Our research team at The Miami Project started to look at the cause of concussions. Collectively, we made a decision to make concussions a primary area of focus.

The more research we did, the more obvious it was that there are serious repercussions to playing football. Adam Goldstein is president of Royal Caribbean Cruise Line. His son David experienced numerous concussions as a high school soccer player in Miami. As a result,

David started having neurological issues such as headaches and mental acuity and cognitive difficulties that disrupted his education.

David and his father, along with The Miami Project, petitioned the State of Florida legislature to begin baseline studies and mandatory testing of high school athletes in Florida. Players now have to be tested every season as a prerequisite to playing any sport where a head injury could occur. Because of the Goldsteins' efforts, Florida became one of the first states to implement mandatory impact studies.

Over time, the discussion about concussions began to dominate media headlines. The ever-increasing appearance of concussion-related problems directed questions to the NFL, specifically to what degree the league knew or should have known the long-term neurological problems associated with playing the game. Initially there was only anecdotal evidence. As an outside observer, I didn't have a direct concern or worry. All the men in my home played football at a high level. We had related aches and pains, but no neurological problems.

That reality ended dramatically and unexpectedly. The problems unfolded over a couple years. My father became to fall down. He had always been clumsy, but this was different. The falls were neither predictable, or particularly often, at least initially. Still, his balance clearly was affected. The falls led to cuts and bruises.

Around the same time, I began to notice that my father would struggle searching for words when we had a conversation. His thoughts were clear, but he was frustrated with the periodic inability to express himself fully. It became painfully clear that he was undergoing some kind of neurological episode. I came to understand and see football as a sport to be feared.

My dad started a journey through the medical industry with the same focus and attention he did for everything in life. He wanted to understand why his condition, of which he remains well aware, continued to worsen. He saw doctors at the University of Miami Miller School, NYU Langone Medical Center, and Ronald Reagan UCLA Medical Center.

The physicians had varying diagnosis but they agreed on one thing: The symptoms were getting worse. I watched an unbreakable icon, a fearless man of action slow down. The transition seemed to begin slowly, and then it happened all at once. It is difficult to watch the physical and psychological deterioration of anyone, but especially for a proud man such as my father. His zest for life, the outward expression of an intense inner drive started to fade away like a setting sun.

My dad accomplished so much. He overcame huge obstacles to become a hero and legend to so many, including me. Nothing came easy, though that never mattered to my dad. They said he was too small for professional football. That's only because they couldn't measure his heart or his mind.

He rose to the top of every profession he entered. He was a highly successful lawyer. He represented a stable of high-profile professional athletes. He became President and Chief Operating Officer of a Fortune 500 company. He hosted the longest running sports show on cable television, *Inside the NFL* on HBO. Then, when he should have been basking in the glow of an incredible life full of accomplishment and adulation, he dedicated himself to helping his son and finding a cure for paralysis.

My father never paid attention to those who said he couldn't do something. As I said in my Hall of Fame speech, maybe my dad was just a poor listener. I do know this: people embrace him. It was a pleasure for nearly everyone who came in contact with my dad to experience a man who an unflinching spirit for life, a passion for excellence, and the fearlessness of a born leader.

I know what the future holds for him. Aside from the continued deterioration, the doctors agree that he will eventually succumb to the neurological problems. It's hard to imagine life without him. He has been, and remains, my best friend.

I owe everything to my dad. I only hope that I have earned a modicum of the respect and admiration I have for him.

For years, I thought that the chance of having a debilitating injury was worth the risk given all the benefits of team sports. The Buonicontis owe a lot to the game of football. I can honestly say that I can attribute a lot of my recovery to what I learned on the football field. The training, the preparation, the hand-to-hand combat, and the nature of a physical game that tested toughness and teamwork on every play—all of that has informed my life since my injury.

Now, however, I can no longer encourage young athletes to play football. If I had a son, I would not allow him to play. Parents should think long and hard about whether or not playing the game is in the best interests of their children. It has been proven that contact sports can produce permanent brain damage.

Chapter 62

Carpe Diem

I never tried to rationalize my injury. I never asked why. That question was never why I got down or depressed. I keep an eye on the future, and not much differently from the way I've lived my entire life, I live for the day. I'm not sure how many days I have. There are so many complications that I face on a daily basis that it doesn't pay to look too far down the road. Many people utter this expression, but I truly do live for the day.

I try to find the happiness in daily life, enjoying the simple moments. I don't need to go out and look for happiness. I'm at peace with myself in my own mind. The things I like to do now involve going out of my way for someone else.

It's not about *me* anymore. That was a long time ago. I like to do for others. It's fun. It's enriching. But I like to go out of my way and do it beyond the normal expectation.

Look at all the outpouring of love and support I have received and continue to receive. I'm just trying to pay it back. I relish their joy. For instance, take money. I don't understand anybody who has millions of dollars, who then waits until they are dead to give it away. Give it away while you are alive and luxuriate in the joy you are able to bring to others. Leaving it in a will? What's the point? You're dead. It's too late then.

I try to not involve myself in unnecessary negative thoughts. Life is too beautiful. Today was beautiful. I went outside and had lunch. It was nothing more than eating and talking with friends out in the sun. I'd be content with the rest of my life filled with days like that.

If I die tomorrow, I can honestly say I'm happy. I have enjoyed my life, and no one can tell me I haven't. Hopefully, along the way, I've also brought some joy to other people's lives. Yes, in the past I brought quite a bit of misery to some people, particularly my mother. I hope I've made amends for those actions more than any others. Everyone can help someone. Ironically, despite my paralysis, I probably have more opportunity to help others, which is reason alone to do so.

People live with blinders on. They never stop and just look around. I absorb life. I have always been an active participant in it. I'm not just passing through. Believe it or not, I enjoy my life as much today as I ever have.

It's still hard talking to individuals who have just become paralyzed or have suffered a brain injury. It brings back all the memories of what I have been through. But I do what I can because I know it's the right thing to do. I know I can provide at least some level of comfort just from my experience.

Then there is Ashley. She was seven years old and sitting in the front seat of her mother's car. Her mother stopped at a stop sign. Another car collided into theirs going less than ten miles an hour. The air bag went off, and the force of the releasing bag broke Ashley's neck. The break was at C1, the top of her spine, and she has been a quadriplegic and on a respirator ever since. That little girl never had a chance in life. She will be on a respirator for the rest of her life and yet she plows ahead, making a real life for herself.

The first time we met was at a restaurant. Ashley was nine or ten at the time and just so precious and beautiful. We started a friendship, and we have been close ever since. I would go over to her house for family barbecues. I've been fortunate enough to watch her grow into a beautiful young woman. I went to her high school graduation and cheered her on as she graduated from college.

She currently works at The Miami Project. She remains an inspiration and a beacon of light for everyone who has the pleasure of knowing her. She is one of my biggest heroes and the reason The Miami Project exists, to give a second chance to people who need it most.

It took a broken neck to slow me down, to ground me. In retrospect that's what it took for me to channel all the passion, energy, drive, and curiosity that made me who I was, into the person I have become.

My spirit, tenacity, and zest for life never changed. It's just been transferred to another life.

Chapter 63

A Day in the Life

The start of the day is the only aspect of my life that is normal compared to the average person. When I open my eyes for the first time in the morning I usually gather my thoughts. I think about what the day ahead has in store. I don't have to sleep on my back, but I do. After a few minutes of contemplation, I call out to my nurse through an intercom system connected to his room. My nurse comes in and opens the blackout shades covering the windows.

He removes sheets and blankets, and then inflates the air mattress on my select-comfort bed. By the way, my sleep number is 35. He pulls the corners of the bed sheets up to free them from the mattress. Then he stands at the foot of the bed and pulls the sheets toward him, which edges my body forward so that my legs hang off the foot of the bed. Having done that, he puts a firm foam wedge behind my back, which forces me into a sitting position. Then he bends my legs up and slides a pad up under my torso. Once those elements are secured, he lifts one of my legs to insert two suppositories into my rectum.

In the half-hour it takes for the suppositories to work, two things happen. First, my nurse catheterizes me to drain my urine. Then I have a breakfast that consists of about a dozen or so spoonsful of dry cereal, either Wheaties or Go-Lean. I don't use milk because it's much easier and quicker just to eat out of the box.

After breakfast, my nurse cleans and disinfects my urine drainage bags. I use two different urine collection bags, one for daytime and one for evening. The morning version is a 1200 cc bag that's connected to my leg via a strap below one knee. The bag is connected to a tube that runs up my thigh and into an external catheter condom. Because I urinate frequently, the bag must be completely emptied several times during the day.

With a few minutes to spare before the suppositories begin to work, my nurse takes my vital signs. That process includes taking my blood pressure, pulse rate, temperature, and so on, as part of a morning assessment. The suppositories begin to take effect, and my nurse transfers me to my waterproof shower/commode chair. After I've had a bowel movement, I head into the shower, which is one of the most rewarding and relaxing moments of my day. My daily shower is like a form of meditation. I usually sit under the water for at least thirty minutes before I actually start soaping up. The sensation that comes from sitting under hot water is like an automatic stress release. Due to my injury, the places on my body where I still have feeling are hypersensitive. I sit right under the shower head. The water is hotter than normal, which in turn soothes my muscles. Eventually my nurse washes my body and shampoos my hair. By the time my shower is finished I've been awake for two and a half hours.

After I'm dried off, I am transferred back to bed so I can be dressed. That takes another forty-five minutes and includes another transfer, this one from the bed to my power chair. It takes roughly three and a half hours from the moment I open my eyes until I'm ready to face the day.

Three days a week, in addition to my shower routine, I have physical and occupational therapy at home.

Then it's off to work. By the time I reach The Miami Project's offices it's noon. Between prescriptions and supplements, I take at least twenty pills throughout the course of the day. One condition common among quadriplegics is low core body temperature due to the lack of circulation and the autonomic dysfunction. The best way to explain the situation is that quadriplegics are cold-blooded animals as compared to the average warm-blooded person. We are like reptiles. Our body temperature is regulated by the surrounding environment. When alligators are warm, they enter the water to cool their bodies. When they're cold, they sun themselves on the shore. Quadriplegics are the same. Whenever I'm in a cool room or outside on a cold day, my body temperature drops significantly. The same thing happens in reverse. For me, it's always a struggle to stay warm, which is telling because I live in South Florida.

One way I regulate my body temperature is by drinking hot water, a common practice of quadriplegics. Even my friends are prepared when they come over to my house because the temperature never goes below seventy-six degrees. Quite often, my sliding door is open to allow the warm, humid air to circulate inside.

Throughout the day, constant adjustments and procedures are part of my routine. For example, catheterizing to empty my bladder every five hours. Reclining my wheelchair to release the pressure on my body to reduce the possibility of getting a decapodous ulcer—a pressure sore—which can be a significant medical complication. Left untreated those ulcers can be life- threatening. That's exactly what killed Christopher Reeve.

I have frequent muscle spasms that are generally controlled but at times can be disconcerting. My chronic bronchitis is always a concern. Not to mention, my lung capacity due to my injury has been weakened to 25 percent of normal. My nurses perform chest physiotherapy to loosen any mucus that might inhibit my breathing and help me cough.

I drink at least three liters of water every day. Even though I catheterize every five hours, sometimes I urinate on my own. I had a sphincterotomy performed that allows easier urine flow when the bladder contracts. Even with that procedure, when my bladder contracts my body experiences episodes of autonomic dysreflexia, which I explained earlier. Once again, it's a dangerous condition and, if not treated immediately, can be fatal.

No matter where I go or what I do, this routine is part of my everyday life. Between work and social activities, appearances, and meetings, my day usually doesn't end until midnight and sometimes later.

The only other part of my day that resembles that of an average person is when I finally go to bed. But even then, I am fitted with a BiPAP machine in order to keep my lungs inflated during the night as a result of my sleep apnea, not to mention a number of other potential complications. I go through the process of being undressed, lifted out of my chair, and put in bed. If I become too warm, or too cold in the middle of the night, I have to wake my nurse so that covers can be removed or added. I might have an itch. I might get something in my eye. Anything can pop up, but there isn't anything I can personally do about it.

One of the best things about going to sleep is that in my dreams, I walk.

Chapter 64

Cynthia

Going back to my grandfather and inclusive of my uncles, father, and brother, Buoniconti men have a deep appreciation for, and attraction to, women. A lot of things changed after my injury. My connection to women was not one of them.

With that said, I always had tremendous difficulty remaining faithful to girlfriends. Part of it has to do with Miami. I put Miami at the top of the list for having the most beautiful women in the world. Not California, New York, or even Rio de Janeiro compares to the diversity of beauty in Miami. There are so many beautiful women that I practically fall in love every day.

In high school I thought I was a gigolo. In actuality, I was just a cocky and conceited kid who saw value only in opportunity rather than in the benefits of commitment and fidelity. I dated girls from three different high schools at the same time. I was trying to be a playboy, selfishly enjoying everything that Miami had to offer in the early '80s, which was a lot.

One of the weekend hotspots in those days was Sundays on the Bay—an outdoor bar on Key Biscayne, just southeast of downtown Miami. My crew and I were there every weekend. We had friends who worked the door, waited tables, and bartended. Getting in underage wasn't an issue, and the Rum Runners flowed abundantly and—let's just say, inexpensively—always with a Bacardi 151 "floater" to boot.

Frequently I went with my buddy Rick Arango, who later became the Obsession model for Calvin Klein. Needless to say, he was eye candy for all the girls. That was part of my MO. I knew the girls would be looking at Rick, so, like a remora attached to a shark, I hung around him. For all his good looks, Rick didn't have the gift of gab. That's where I earned my stripes. We scoped out different pairs of girls. Then I would use my communication skills to break the ice. I'd approach the girls and say, "That's my friend over there. He'd really like to meet you." And the deal was sealed.

A lot of "firsts" took place at my friend Dodie's house. It wasn't because his parents didn't care what we did. It's just that they spent a lot of weekends away at their house in Hollywood Beach, Florida. Actually, most everything worth happening during those years happened at Dodie's. It's where I got drunk for the first time. It's where I smoked pot for the first time. About the only thing I didn't do for the first time at Dodie's was lose my virginity.

That happened when I was fifteen years old. I heard about this girl who had a reputation for being promiscuous. My good friend Charlie was dating one of her friends, a girl I've known since first grade. I told Charlie to set me up with them on a double date. We started the night at a point at the end of a long road in a community called Gables by the Sea, where we drank a bottle of Mumm champagne. Then we drove to an empty lot behind nearby Gulliver Academy. Everyone has a story of the first time. That is mine.

At the beginning of my sophomore year at The Citadel, I began dating a girl who I knew from Coral Gables High. She happened to be starting her freshman year at the College of Charleston. Of course, relationships were difficult at The Citadel because cadets are confined to campus during the week. I couldn't stay out overnight on the weekends either because I was always on restriction.

However, I often went AWOL during my sophomore year. I asked one of my classmates to temporarily sleep in my bed when officers checked rooms before lights out. Or if the guy doing the checking was a friend, I'd let him know what was going on so he wouldn't turn me in. That was the only way I could get an overnight away from campus.

After my injury, I was concerned about whether or not I could ever have sex again. As I mentioned earlier, I can't not move my arms or my legs, but I can achieve an erection.

One of the guys I met in rehab had been recently discharged and was staying at a hotel right across the street from the rehab center. In the summer of 1986, less than a year after my injury, the girl I dated in Charleston came home for the summer. After a few days of visits, it was time to take our interaction to the next level. I secured a connecting room at the hotel. I told her that I needed to lay down for a little while to get the pressure off my butt. I think she knew that I was just trying to get alone with her. Anyway, let's just say that it was a wonderful afternoon. To this day, we are friends. I will always be thankful to her for helping me achieve a huge milestone in my psychological and physical recovery. That experience allowed me to have the confidence to explore other relationships and begin that next chapter of my life.

One of my favorite restaurants in Miami was a Thai restaurant called Siam Palace. I went there for the first time in 1996 with one of my ex-girlfriends. The food at Siam Palace was absolutely delicious, and it was a great place to take girls out to dinner. The owner, Cynthia, was always very nice and extremely professional, not to mention incredibly beautiful.

Early on I inquired about her to one of the servers, who informed me that she was married. I just left it at that. For the next twelve years, I went to Siam Palace about twice a month. During that time, I dated a lot of different girls. I took nearly all of them to Siam Palace. Little did I know that I was the subject of a lot of banter among the staff, including Cynthia, who considered me to be a serial philanderer.

Then, in October 2007, I went to Siam Palace with a girl that I was dating. Right as I rolled in, Cynthia greeted me and promptly sat us at my regular table. There was something different about her that night. As I mentioned, she's a beautiful woman, but it was more than that. She was glowing. I couldn't keep my eyes off of her. I felt sorry for my date because I really didn't pay much attention to her during the dinner. All my attention was on Cynthia. I was mesmerized.

The feeling was so strong I returned for lunch a few days later. She was so busy running around the restaurant it was hard to engage her in any meaningful conversation. So I came up with a plan: I called Cynthia and told her that I wanted her restaurant to cater my annual New Year's Eve party.

She must have thought I was crazy because I called so many times to make adjustments to the menu. It was the only way I could meet with her again. I always ordered some food to go, and I asked Cynthia to walk me out. During one of the walks, I found out that she was separated from her husband.

I invited her to a Buoniconti Fund event, but she was noncommittal. But on our little walk to my car I said, "I am really enjoying getting to know you. I am happy that we are becoming friends." She followed by saying, "Me too, as long as we stay friends."

For any guy, being referred to as a "friend" is the kiss of death. I remember saying to myself, "Okay, stop pursuing her, she sent you a message loud and clear." I stopped calling, and visiting the restaurant. Then, one evening, while attending the event she had turned down my invitation to, I received a call on my mobile phone. The caller ID read, *Cynthia*.

"Hello Cynthia, how are you?"

"Oh my God, I called the wrong Mark," she said.

"No, you called the right Marc!"

"I was trying to call my dishwasher, whose name is Mark."

We said our goodbyes, but all I thought was, "Sure she was trying to call her dishwasher." It was just an excuse to call me because she realized that I stopped calling and visiting. Rather than give up, I took the "misdial" as a hint to continue the courtship.

The following week I had lunch at her restaurant, and on our walk back to the car I flat out asked her to lunch at my condo. She accepted. It was Friday, April 11, and we had a beautiful afternoon. We took a little walk down by the pool to a secluded seating area under a tree. We talked a little more, then I asked her for a hug. What started out as a harmless little hug, turned into the most passionate, romantic, and unforgettable kiss of my life. Well, as they say, the rest is history, and we've been together ever since.

Cynthia truly is the most incredible woman I've ever met. All I ever wanted was a woman who loved me as much as I loved her. That's exactly what we have together. I know it sounds cliché, but she truly makes me want to be a better man. We have dedicated our lives to each other, and there's nothing I wouldn't do in this world for her. She is incredibly caring and selfless when it comes to taking care of me. We are the epitome of two people in love, who are also each other's best friend. You might be asking: If you two are so in love, then why aren't you married? The reason is as simple as it is absurd.

When I was injured in 1985, my father was working for U.S. Tobacco. He had the foresight to make sure that my brother and I were covered by the company's catastrophic insurance policy. For more than thirty years that fateful decision has kept me alive. However, the policy states that I must remain single and financially dependent on my father. It's true, I am dependent on my father, but even if I were married, I would remain dependent on my father because he is the life-long conduit to the policy. I don't know why the insurance company would care whether I was married. It wouldn't affect the costs associated with my care. It's crazy.

With that said, I cannot jeopardize my insurance by getting married. But the technicality didn't keep me from making the kind of commitment to Cynthia that she deserves. On the evening of October 24, 2011, while enjoying a specially prepared meal and the romantic sounds of a harpist, I proposed. Through tears of joy she accepted.

For now, Cynthia and I will remain happily engaged, having promised to be together forever, knowing in our hearts that we are soul mates.

Chapter 65

Tick Tock

Through the grace of God, and the around-the-clock nursing care available to me, I have remained relatively healthy for more than thirty years. Of course, and as expected, there have been several bumps along the road, including surgeries and dozens of procedures. I've survived life-threatening infections, blood clots, and numerous other near-death experiences, many of them recounted here previously.

The most problematic and ongoing medical concern is urinary tract infections (UTIs). For a majority of us with spinal cord injuries, dealing with UTIs is a constant and unrelenting problem.

Due to my injury, I don't have voluntary control of the sphincter muscle in and around the bladder neck. Those muscles enable the bladder to open and close to facilitate urination. That means I am unable to empty my bladder normally, which results in high residuals of urine remaining in the bladder. Over time those residuals become stagnant. The result is a robust breeding ground for bacteria. Virtually every person with spinal cord injury endures the threat and effects of UTIs.

Kidney stones are another problem that contributes to UTIs. Bacteria grow within, and hide inside, the stones, and are impervious to antibiotics. Kidney stone infections beget a vicious cycle. I can take an antibiotic treatment for a UTI. Then once I stop taking the antibiotics I am re-infected by the bacteria in the stones. The worst part, of course, is that over time the bacteria become antibiotic resistant. That's why a UTI can kill a person with a spinal cord injury. Antibiotic resistance sets the stage for super infections and eventual death from septicemia. The body simply becomes overwhelmed by the infection.

I am often asked what it's like being confined to a wheelchair. The wheelchair is the easiest part. The hard part is complications, which are ever-present. Over time, the UTIs create chronic problems, any one of which can kill me. As I said, I am susceptible to kidney stones, bladder cancer, and kidney disease.

Due to the high level of my injury, my breathing remains significantly compromised. A minor chest cold can turn into full-blown pneumonia. It is a constant struggle to keep my lungs clear.

The risk of a skin ulcer is a daily concern, as well. My nurses and I are extremely vigilant when it comes to my skin, which is always at risk of breaking down.

Sitting in a wheelchair sixteen hours a day for more than thirty years has taken a toll on my spine. Scoliosis, a curvature of the spine, is a given. Not standing makes my bones decalcify, which causes osteoporosis and can lead to bone fractures and further complications. I take calcium supplements that include vitamin D to replace calcium and ward off different cancers.

Despite all the precautions and around-the-clock nurses, I wasn't prepared for what happened in February 2014.

All I remember is opening my eyes and staring at the ceiling, realizing that I was back on a respirator in the hospital with no recollection of the what, where, when, or how. The only thing I knew was that the "who" was me, and it didn't look good.

It was like returning to a nightmare. I couldn't talk, so instinctively I started clicking my mouth and tongue in an attempt to get someone's attention. Unbeknownst to me, Cynthia and my mother were sitting at my side. They jumped up, happy to see me awake.

I mouthed "What happened?" and "Where am I?" They told me that six days earlier I had been complaining of a strange sensation, like a bone floating in and around my chest cavity. I was admitted to the hospital on Thursday, February 26, 2014. It was determined that my gallbladder needed to be removed. The surgery went fine. That night due to a combination of the anesthesia, pain medication, and an undiagnosed case of sleep apnea, I wasn't breathing well. To make matters worse, I told all the nurses and staff not to bother me so I could get some badly needed rest. Throughout the night my breathing wasn't deep enough to maintain normal oxygen levels. That caused a dangerous rise in my carbon dioxide levels. Eventually the carbon dioxide became toxic and rendered me unconscious.

Fortunately, the nursing staff ignored the request to leave me alone. At 6 a.m. they entered my room to do a routine assessment, only they couldn't wake me. The nurses immediately called a code blue, which in medical terms means respiratory arrest. Within minutes I was intubated and connected to a respirator, but I was far from out of the woods. By then, Dr. Green arrived and took over.

I was told that the team shook me—continuously. I remained unresponsive. Then, as I was being prepared to be transferred into the ICU, I went into convulsions. My nurse, Peter, called Cynthia, who raced to the hospital. She called my father and my friend Dodie.

Cynthia sat by my bedside as they worked to revive me, but my father couldn't deal with the frenzy and my condition. He waited outside my room. There were a dozen doctors, nurses, and technicians involved. Once I was intubated, I became stable enough to be moved to the neurological intensive care unit, just a couple of floors above.

It's reasonable to assume that recovery comes quicker in the ICU. Not in my case. Twice doctors tried to remove the respirator. Each time my oxygen levels deteriorated rapidly. My cough reflex was so weak that I was unable to clear my lungs. Unable to survive off the respirator, I developed pneumonia and my lungs began to collapse. If there was a silver lining, it was that I was oblivious.

I was admitted to the hospital on a Thursday, had surgery on Friday, crashed and nearly died on Saturday. I didn't wake up until the following Wednesday. When I did, I looked around and basically freaked out.

In the words of Yogi Berra, it was *déjà vu* all over again.

Once again, I had no choice. I had to figure out a path to recovery. The first goal was to improve my respiratory status, clear the pneumonia, and pump up my lungs. It took weeks of lung suctioning, chest physiotherapy, and strengthening my body before the respirator was removed. It was a struggle. Every time the respirator was about to be removed, my lungs collapsed, filling up with secretions, and the process started all over again.

It became a neverending roller coaster of emotions and physical breakdowns. Finally, they decided to try to remove the respirator one more time. Initially, I was doing fine. But within hours, secretions started to build up. I was unable to create a productive cough. My lungs filled. That evening as I struggled to breathe, they intubated me again. I was more depressed than fearful.

Weeks went by. If I couldn't breathe on my own, then the next step was surgery for a tracheotomy. That meant the insertion of a semipermanent plastic tube down my throat. It would be a conduit for the respirator.

They decided to give me one more chance.

My father suggested a bronchoscopy, which employs a mechanically operated suction machine deep inside the lungs. The premise was that if I got a good cleaning, then there would be less secretion that I had to push out myself. If it worked, I had a better chance of staying off the respirator.

When the time came to attempt to remove the respirator one last time, I was terrified. The process is extremely uncomfortable. It left my throat sore and raw. Once it was removed, I had to be able to cough up secretions on my own. Eventually, I was able to mobilize the secretions and expel them. It's hard to explain how monumental it was, yet again, to be free of the respirator.

A week later I was transferred to the step-down unit, which is a less intensive hospital room where I remained monitored.

That's when it was decided that I would need to use a BiPAP machine in the evening to deal with my sleep apnea and to keep my lungs open and oxygenated. It was a small price to pay given the alternatives: a tracheotomy or a permanent resting place six feet under.

Still, there was significant anxiety and uncertainty when I was sent home. I had endured another brush with death, the closest one since the initial days following my injury. I wanted to go home, but there is a sense of security that comes from all the care and technology that kept me alive in the hospital. The security blanket was gone. Even though I knew my nurses and Cynthia would be by my side, a heightened sense of concern remained in the back of my mind.

I never imagined that I would have to face the grueling experience of being back on a respirator. Once again, I had to muster every bit of life energy in order to preserve my quality of life.

Thanks to incredible medical care, a strong support system, and through the grace of God, I made it back home again. In some respects, I was stronger than I had been in years.

It's true what they say. Whatever doesn't kill you makes you stronger.

* * *

DAD: Marc was like most normal sixteen- to nineteen-year-olds growing up. Since his injury, his transformation has been remarkable. He has become a leader. He has become a defender for people with disabilities. He's shown an incredible ability to smile when most people would cry. He is courageous because every day that he wakes up his arms and legs don't move. Yet he pushes on throughout the day.

He's eloquent. He's handsome. He still loves women. There may be a lot of things that don't work, but his eyes work fine.

In the final analysis when everything is said and done, when people are getting out of wheelchairs and walking, hugging people and loving people and doing things they never thought they'd ever be able to do again, they really will have one person to thank. That's Marc.

He has driven himself to be the poster boy for spinal cord injury. He won't rest until people are walking or function is restored.

It's remarkable to me how he is able to carry himself the way he does every day. I say that not as Marc's father, but just as an observer of a quadriplegic. Every day it's got to be the most difficult, torturous effort to get out of bed and get on with your life and help push the program forward. It's easy for me to say, but he's such a courageous guy.

Marc would have had a turnaround because something would have forced him to turn his life around. The life he was leading as a young man was not the life he was capable of leading.

He has so much going for himself. He has such a great intellect. He would have been a great politician. He could have been governor of the state of Florida. He could have been anything he wanted to be. He's got that much intelligence, drive, and charisma.

Chapter 66

The Power That Moves Me

What is it about tragedy that elicits the best from many of us? Perhaps it's the emotion that is dragged to the surface that forces us into the present moment. The intensity demands attention, and awareness is thrust upon us.

I have been in a wheelchair for far more years than I was able to move. Despite countless challenges across the human spectrum—emotional, physical, and spiritual—paralysis didn't merely save my life. The hardship produced a depth of life I couldn't have imagined otherwise. It's a remarkable statement, I know. But I found my humanity. The same spirit that drove me to achieve on the football field and fueled the free-range life I lived is the same one that informed my rebirth—in a wheelchair.

My injury revealed to me a burning desire to dedicate my life to helping others, including, but not limited to, finding a cure for paralysis. Ten seconds before I collapsed on a football field in Tennessee—unable to move, barely able to sustain enough breath to save myself— not even I could have imagined the person I would become. In an instant I was forced to confront myself beyond the context of my athletic prowess, much less my interests. Who I had been was not going to be who I was destined to become.

I had a choice, as all of us do when confronted with catastrophic change. I had to go inside myself to find a way back into the world. I could have given up. Who would have blamed me if I had? Who could have blamed my father for accepting what was considered, at the time, settled science? It's in the darkest hour, when courage is nearly depleted and hope is nothing more than a word that giving up is most seductive. That's not how life-changing moments are defined, though. We know that because no one recalls those who gave in and gave up. What we remember are those who dared to move forward with dignity even amid great uncertainty.

I'm reminded of my late friend Muhammad Ali, who said:

"Impossible is just a word thrown around by small men who find it easier to live in the world they've been given than to explore the power they have to change it. Impossible is not a fact. It's an opinion. Impossible is potential. Impossible is temporary. Impossible is nothing."

My father made a promise that started with his son, but it extended to everyone in a wheelchair at the time and those who would be in a wheelchair in the future. It was more than the selfless act of a grieving father. It was transformative for me. My life-changing moment occurred due to a collision on a football field. My life changed from catastrophic injury to recovery when my dad looked into my eyes and promised to make a difference. To know my father was to know that he would not rest until he had found a way forward.

I couldn't allow him to take such a journey on my behalf without being alongside him.

Life presents hardships to everyone usually at the same time it offers a unique opportunity to define who we are against who we might become. I'm not sure when, how, or if I would have become the person I am without being forced to change my perspective on life. I was awakened. Shaken and challenged to be sure, but all in the process of becoming clear about what is and is not important. I wish I could move just enough to feed myself. I wish I could put my arms around Cynthia. I wish I could stand, even for a minute each day.

Would I trade it all for the life I was leading a little over thirty years ago? Not if it meant erasing what I have experienced as a result of my injury. I learned to take nothing for granted. I learned what it feels like to be dedicated to people and circumstances beyond my own interests. I learned a lot about myself, much of which I didn't like. I hurt a lot of people. I made bad choices. My injury provided an opportunity to make amends, to clean the slate so that I could move forward in good standing with God and myself.

I know my obligation to society. I was given a second chance. I was able to experience the true measure of a man by watching my father dedicate the second half of his adult life to his son, and on behalf of people he would never meet.

We all have the opportunity to find meaning amid the madness of life. A catastrophe forces the issue, but it's not necessary.

Look inside.

Find your passion.

Embrace your potential.

Get involved.

Selflessness and altruism are their own rewards.

When you look back on your life, be the person that makes you proud.

ACKNOWLEDGEMENTS

A special thank you to all the people who helped me throughout my journey. It is because of all of you that I am the person that I am today.

Cynthia Vijitakula

Teresa Buoniconti & George "Chris" Pedersen

Nicholas A. Buoniconti & Lynn Buoniconti

Nicholas A. Buoniconti III & Dena

Gina Bruce

Nicholas Buoniconti IV

Gabriela Bruce

Sophia Buoniconti

Danielle Bruce

Robert & Candice Buoniconti

Peter & Joanne Buoniconti

Michael Buoniconti

Vincent & Meg Buoniconti

Barth A. Green, MD, FACS & Kathy L. Green

Pond-Radee "Win" Halelamien

Edward & Eileen Salamano

Miami Dolphins

1982 Christopher Columbus State Final Football Team

Citadel F Troop Classmates

Bal Harbour Shops

Bal Harbour Village

Barton G

The Buoniconti Fund Board of Trustees

The Buoniconti Fund Chapters

The Collection

Diageo

Southern Wine and Spirits

Tiffany & Co.

United Airlines

HBO

Maloney & Porcelli Quality Branded

New York Hilton Midtown

Waldorf Astoria New York City

George Abaunza, PhD

Gary Abramson

Alexandre Abreu, MD

Gisela Aguila Puentes, MD

Richard S. Aldrich, Jr.

Dick Anderson

Jamie Anderson

Ron Anderson

Enrique Arango

Teresa D. Arcay

Micky & Madeleine Arison

Gayle Balth

Louis F. Bantle

Robert C. Bantle

Candice Barrs

Gregory W. Basil, MD

William Beckham

Woody Beckham

Teri Bendell-Bou

Jim and Maddie Berlin

Diana Berning

Scott Bistrong

Sylvia Bistrong

Ronald Bogue

Ron L. Book, Esq.

Richard R. Booth

Romero Britto

Ina W. Broeman

Tom Brokaw

Richard Bunge, MD

Mary Bunge, PhD

James M. Callahan, Sr.

Carter Burrus, PhD

Jimmy Cahill

Robert Cahill

Jerry Callahan

Skip Campbell

Lydia Cannady (Hollister, Inc.)

Diana Cardenas, MD

Eileen Carey (Hollister, Inc.)

Adam E. Carlin

Randy Carlson

Harry Carson

Richard D. Catenacci, Esq.

Christina Chambers Gilfillan

Raymond G. Chambers

Alexander Chudnoff

Charles Cinnamon

Robin Cleary

President William "Bill" Clinton

Linda Coll

John Conomikes

Bob Costas

Wendy Crawford

Mark F. Dalton

Eddie Dauer

Scott DeNight

George Dennis

Congressman Mario Diaz-Balart

Col. Harvey M. Dick (The Citadel)

Dalton W. Dietrich, PhD

Swanee & Paul DiMare

Kevin Dufford

Frank Eismont, MD

Lenore Elias

Rudy Eljaiek, BA ATP

Wendy Elkin

Gloria and Emilio Estefan

Chris Evert

Rudy Fernandez

State Attorney Katherine
    Fernandez-Rundle

James Ferraro

Emerson Fittipaldi

Edward Thaddeus "Tad" Foote
    (Past President of U of M)

Julio Frenk, MD

James Gabrish

Tim Gannon

Honorable Judge Barry L.
    & Bobbi Garder

Shelley Garcia, RN

Betty Gardner

Jose Garrido, MD

Joe Gaskins

Pascal Goldschmidt, MD

Christopher Gomez, MD

Evelyn Gomez

Henry Gonzalez

Sergio M. Gonzalez

Ken Gorin

John Gray

Richard W. Gray

Ross Greenberg

Darrell Gwynn

Brother Kevin Handibode

Tim Hanlon

Thomas J. Harrington, MD

J. Ira Harris

Alan F. & Connie Herbert
  (Hollister, Inc.)

Jerry Herbst

John Hess

Commissioner Sally A. Heyman

Bea Hollfelder

Scott Holloway (Hollister, Inc.)

Lester Holt

Thomas Hooten, MD

Harry Horgan

Wayne Huizenga

Carlos Ibietatorremendia

Julio Iglesias

Chuck Jackson

Ira Jacobson, MD

Billy Jenkinson

Paul Tudor Jones

Rich Jones

Tommy Lee & Dawn Jones

Jay Jordan

Roger King

Mike Kissenberth

Kevin Kitchmefsky

Philip H. Knight

Debra Koch

Jeffrey Kramer

Kandy Kramer

Jon Krupnick

Howard Landi, MD

Kirk Landon

Edie Laquer

Senator Jack Latvala

Thomas J. LeBlanc, PhD

Nathan H. Lebwohl, MD

Tova Leidesdorf

James R. Leininger, MD

Raymond Leveillee, MD

Allan Levi, MD, PhD, FAC

Richard L. Levine, MD

Christine E. Lynn

Charles Lynne, MD

Martin Maddaloni

George V. Malickel (Hollister, Inc)

Kelly Mallette

Richard Manz

Jacqueline Manzano

Ashley Moore Marcucci

Alberto Martinez-Arizala, MD

Mead McCabe

John McCannon

Randy Medendwall

Deborah Mellon

Carlos Migoya

Stuart Miller

Donald Misner

Keith Misner

Jim Monahan

David Moore

Nat Moore

Elizabeth Morra

Diana Morrison

Michael Morgan

Peter Morton

Senator Bill Nelson

Jack & Barbara Nicklaus

President Richard M. Nixon

Craig Nielsen

Patrick Noble (Hollister, Inc.)

Dottie and Henry Norton

Steven Olvey, MD

Kristine H. O'Phelan, MD

John Osterweil

Ricky Palermo

James J. Pallotta

Judy Pantoja and Mead McCabe

Angel Pardo (DMR)

Joyce and Louis Park

Tony Podesta

Steven Petrillo

William Pearson

Lois Pope

Stewart Rahr

Ivelisse Raimundi, PhD

Victoria Ranger Nunez

Carole Robbins

Lt. Gen. John Rosa (The Citadel)

Beth Roscoe

Scott Roy

Ethan Ruby

Abbey Ruttenberg

Bill Ryan Jr.

Bill Ryan Sr.

Matthis Salathe, MD

Morris Sands, MD

Suzanne M. Sayfie

Eugene Sayfie, MD

Stephanie Sayfie-Aagaard

Daniel Schleifman

John A. Schneider

Jeremy Schwartz

Ake Seiger, MD

Donna E. Shalala

Patrick Sheehy

Coach Don Shula

Senator Ron Silver

William A. Simon

Daniel Sleeman, MD

Bryan Slomovitz, MD

John Stephens

Cheryl Stephenson

Tibor and Hana Stern

Alan N. Stillman

William Stokkan

John Sullivan

Craig Swanson

Bob Tahill

Matthew Telepman

Jacqueline Tommasino

President Donald J. Trump

Marvin Tucker

Steven Vanni, MD

Nicholas J. Verbitsky

Thomas J. Vigorito

Cliff Walters

Adam Wanner, MD

Allison Ward

Marcela Ward

Jo and John Watkins

Barton G. Weiss

UNDEFEATED

Jay Weiss
Kristin Wherry
Randy Whitman
Stanley Whitman
Matthew Whitman Lazenby

Lancelot Williams
Ralph Wilson
Peter D. Winder
Robert C. Wright